FABULOUS YOU!

UNLOCK YOUR PERFECT PERSONAL STYLE

Tori Hartman

Berkley Books, New York

FABULOUS YOU!

A Berkley Book / published by arrangement with
the author

PRINTING HISTORY
Berkley edition / April 1995

ISBN: 0-425-14618-9

BERKLEY®
Berkley Books are published by The Berkley Publishing Group,
200 Madison Avenue, New York, New York 10016.
BERKLEY and the "B" design
are trademarks belonging to Berkley Publishing Corporation.

10   9   8   7   6   5   4   3   2   1

CONTENTS

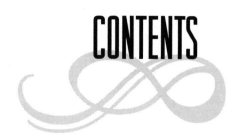

Contents

SECTION III: PUTTING IT ALL TOGETHER   211

Acknowledgments

There are always people who give you support when you're in the creative process. Some by reading, some by critiquing, others by just being there for you. Here are a few of the people I'd like to thank:

KayEllen Bradley, Sharon Carpenter, Jane Carroll, Debbie Corbett, John D'Andrea, Jeff D'Avonso, John Duel, Julie Frankel, Barbara Freeling, Elek Hartman, Joie Karnes, Linda Kelly, Victoria Mahoney, Jeanne Martinet, Maxine Meltzer, Jennifer Merin, Lauren Moon, Susan Schulman.

And a very warm fuzzy to my editor, Elizabeth Beier.

A very special thanks to Carolyn Strauss. Your support and help in creating the Fabulous You! system has been invaluable. You'll always be in style, Tori

INTRODUCTION

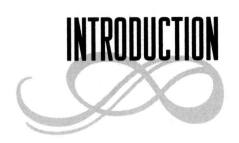

As a child, and later as a teenager, fashion was my nightmare. My mother was very dramatic and a constant confirmation of how bland I felt.

Mom had the ability to walk into a room and seize attention—she was the belle of the ball. Her style always worked on her, and others constantly sought out her wisdom on dressing.

But, alas, for her own daughter, she was an abysmal failure in the makeover department. She resigned herself to the fact that I couldn't wear the flashy things she'd hoped would make us a "team." I was destined to "blend" in. She felt sorry for me; to her, being a "part of" anything was near tragedy. Dramatic people led groups, they didn't join them.

My mother did me a service when she gave up on me. It wasn't until years later that I came to understand that we didn't share a style. Nor did we share the same tastes. I learned that every person has their own natural style type.

But I paid the price of learning. I was mercilessly made fun of by kids in school, teased for having the wrong clothes and the wrong hairstyle. I endlessly searched for a style that would work for me and made some painful mistakes. I sought out dramatic dressers all my life to help spruce me up, and all they ever did was make me look overdone.

In the early 1980s, I began modeling. Since it was a very "classic" time, I finally began to fit in. Clients booked me to model because I had the right "look." I loved modeling because the manufacturers were making clothes somewhere between plain and dazzling, and they worked on me.

By 1985, I finally had something to say about clothing and fit. I was a "petite fashion model" (I'm 5'3"), and other women wanted to know what I had learned in the industry. I began traveling the country and speaking to other women about dressing.

Today I make my living traveling and presenting dressing seminars in department

1

stores. Sales associates frequently are amazed at how willing many of their regular customers are to trust me and buy clothing I suggest.

There are times when I can tell a woman's style just by looking at her. I also know if an associate is showing her customer clothes that she herself likes, but that are not right for the customer's style.

One of the many wonderful sales associates I've met springs to mind. She is what I've labeled a Traditional. She lives in a very traditional area. How successful do you think she is? *Very*. She shows her customers the right looks, and they come back.

As I began to develop my style system, I was able to easily spot a Trendy or Sporty and show them items that would work for them. The women I've worked with began making fewer purchases and enjoying more effective wardrobes. My style system will do the same for you. As you begin to uncover your perfect personal style, you will discover a FABULOUS YOU!

Welcome.

SECTION I

DETERMINING YOUR STYLE

Chapter One

STYLE IS LIFE-STYLE

I'm going to make a bold assumption about you. I'm going to assume you already have a closet full of clothes. And I'm going to assume that you reached for this book not because you necessarily want to buy more for your closet, but to discover how to look your best.

Clients come to me over and over, saying, "I need to *develop* a style." My reply is, let's just *find* your style.

I don't believe that any woman evolves into her style. Or that this, or any book, can help you become a style. I firmly believe that *each* of us is born into one of six style types, which I call: Sporty, Romantic, Traditional, Classic, Dramatic, and Trendy.

Many of us experiment, try to follow trends, or even wear the current "in" outfit. I have nothing against the designers or the trends. But today, we have less and less time to devote to

shopping, and often it's a question of tackling in a few quick hours (if that) the very important task of deciding what we're going to wear for the next six months. We play this hit-or-miss game every season. Imagine your life with fewer fashion mistakes. Imagine a wardrobe of clothing that works for you rather than a few assorted outfits that once made sense to you.

The way to get there is by discovering your *personal style*.

What is it that makes a woman memorable? When it comes to style, I believe what makes someone memorable is congruence. Congruence is when a woman's life matches her style. While Grace Kelly, a stunning Traditional in style, had a thriving career, it was the pull to a more traditional life that created an *unforgettable imprint* on our minds. It was as Princess Grace that she soared.

Truly memorable women are congruent. Imagine Madonna in any role Jane Seymour has played, or vice versa. Madonna is a pure Trendy, able to do her own thing, while Jane Seymour is a Romantic, attached to love and romance. Regardless of what you may think about them, both are quite memorable.

Matching your style to your wardrobe *and* your life will give you the same congruence these memorable women enjoy.

When you learn your own style, you will begin to read the latest trends with a new, educated eye. When fluid fabrics and clothes with movement come onto the scene, for example, Romantics are in their element. Other types may not be. If the look of the season is primarily geared to one style type, other types may have to shop with a more astute eye.

Some designers have their hand on the pulse of the nation—and their styles work for many women. When Liz Claiborne burst onto the scene, her success came from being in touch with women's need for versatility in our wardrobes. Donna Karan identified with our need for fewer pieces that go farther. Every style type can find something in these designers' collections—and the more style types that can wear a designer's goods, the more popular that label becomes.

The problem that most women face is simple to solve: We endlessly search for the outfit or style that suits us, rather than first discovering who we are and what our needs,

likes, and dislikes truly are. Somewhere along the line we get hooked into believing that someone else knows what's best for us. No one knows what's better for you than you do.

Style is more than which belt goes with a particular outfit. Style is life-style. It begins with who you are and how you as an individual would respond to a particular situation. When all of these elements match, you've got congruence!

To unlock your perfect personal style you must remember: **Every woman falls into one of the six style types.**

My friend Kayellen discovered she was a Traditional after she took the style quiz. At first glance, we both thought she was a Romantic. However, after taking the quiz and looking at her life-style, she recognized that her values were more well matched to a Traditional. However, she does have a Romantic accent.

Your accent type is the style type that you easily can borrow a few touches from. Actress Ellen Barkin is a master at this. While she is a Traditional, in movies like *Sea of Love,* she uses Dramatic accents to fill out the role.

Who can deny the instant impression of Candice Bergen as a Classic, or Joan Collins as a Dramatic? How about Julia Roberts as a Sporty? These three women, along with countless others in the spotlight, are all women who have made an impression on us. Why? *Congruence.*

It is the fabulously memorable women in

the world who dress within their style type. You create a strong impact when you do the same.

Our style expresses our individuality. When I first began working with style types, I seriously doubted that my system would work. How could I peg people into a style and then tell them they were unique? It didn't make sense, so I put it aside for a long time. As my career progressed, I came to understand that the parameters of style actually help free women, rather than limit them. The more certain you are of your style, the less likely you are to be fooled by a new trend that absolutely is not you. Isn't that a relief? How would you like to flip through a fashion magazine, absolutely confident of what will work for you and what won't? Once you know your style type, recognizing what is "you" will be simple.

In the individual style type chapters, I give personalized tips and suggestions for each style type. Everyone has an area where they fall down on the "what to wear" front. A Dramatic may know what to wear to the Academy Awards, but send her to an intimate garden wedding and she's lost. Send a Sporty to a formal or semiformal occasion and she's near terror.

There is also the consideration of how fashion forward the city you live in is. I can often determine this by looking at the markdown racks of the local department stores. If the clothes are extremely traditional, it's a fast-paced city. If the clothes are very trendy, I know it's a more traditional town. Whatever *isn't* selling tells me that the women who live there are the opposite.

Quick tip: When traveling to a city that is the opposite of your style type, plan on doing some shopping. You may pick up some great bargains while you're there.

There are times when all of us are intimidated by "fashion" and tend not to like taking chances when dressing, since most of our "risks" have wound up on display at the local thrift shop. We forget the winners because they are few and far between. Once you determine your style, it's a lot harder to make a mistake.

I don't believe that the answer is buying new outfits. It's in reevaluating your needs and updating from there. Much of what you need you probably already own. You don't need much to have a congruent wardrobe, just the ability to edit it into the right pieces for you.

Once we determine your style, we'll integrate all your knowledge of color into a system that makes your daily choices a breeze. My goal is to work all the information you already have into streamlining your wardrobe and making it function for you.

Are you ready to begin?

Like learning any skill, finding your style takes some time. But, if you work through each section (I suggest you do one in its entirety at each sitting), within two weeks you'll be more aware of what makes you look great than you ever believed possible.

STEPS IN DETERMINING YOUR STYLE

1. Take the quiz. It is a written test, and I suggest you set aside at least forty-five minutes to do it properly.
2. Create a collage of your life and style.
3. Write a statement to clarify what you're looking for in your wardrobe.

IMPLEMENTING THE SYSTEM

1. Read the chapter designated for your style and learn about it. I suggest you read the chapter on your accent style as well (that's the style that comes in second in your quiz results).

2. Clean out your closet. It takes longer than going to the dentist, but it's less painful. There is a whole chapter devoted to that, and it will assist you in uncovering your three personal colors, which are vital to building your wardrobe.

3. Study your seasonal color wheel and build your wardrobe using the colors that best reflect who you are and what message you are trying to convey. The Color Glossary is in Chapter Fourteen (page 179), and you can look up the meaning of the colors you choose to wear.

4. The final section of the book is all about the fashion industry and shopping—how, what, when, and where to go. I also give shopping tips and cover special sizes and fit.

Chapter Two

DETERMINING YOUR STYLE — THE QUIZ

The style quiz will take some thinking on your part—thinking like a fashion expert. Please don't underestimate the effectiveness of these questions. Sometimes the silly ones will lend the most insight. That's why I'm not giving you a multiple-choice quiz. Too easy. Besides, everything worth learning takes some effort.

THE STYLE-TYPE QUESTIONNAIRE

Answer the following questions as fully as you can. After you have answered each question, think about a celebrity or someone you admire who would answer the question the same way that you did. Jot down what style type you think *they* could be.

1. Do you use hair spray? Can you think of the brand? Anything particular about it, for example, was it on sale or did it feature certain qualities? Think about what celebrity might also use that same brand.

_____

_____

2. What brands of makeup do you use? Do you favor one brand over the others?

_____

_____

3. For haircuts, do you wait until you can't stand it and then go to the local salon? Or do you go regularly and have one hairdresser?

Do you get the same haircut every time, or a totally different one? Do you trust your hairdresser to do whatever he or she wants?

_____

_____

4. What's your nail-care routine? Do you get manicures regularly, or do them yourself? Do you bite your nails? Are they short or long?

_____

_____

5. What heel height do you prefer in your shoes? Do you have mostly flats or heels? Are all your shoes black, white, or taupe? Or do you have some colors? Is there a brand name that you buy? Is there a style you favor? Strappy sandals, closed pump, sneaker, loafer?

_____

_____

6. Do you buy a name brand of panty hose? Do you buy colors, patterns? Do you like tights? Socks? Do you go without?

_____

_____

7. Regarding undergarments:
   a) Do you wear shoulder pads? How important are they?

   _____

   _____

   b) What style bras do you wear? Any name brands? Do you have all nude/white bras, or do you have red, black, etc? Are they sexy or practical?

   _____

   _____

   c) What style panties do you wear? Sexy or practical? What are the brand names? Colors?

   _____

   _____

   d) Do you wear slips? This one will tell you a lot, so answer it thoroughly.

   _____

   _____

   e) Do you wear nightgowns? Nightshirts? An old T-shirt?

   _____

   _____

8. Is there a designer you like the most?

_____

_____

9. Do you exercise regularly? Is there a sport you like to play?

_____

_____

10. What in your life are you most passionate about?

_____

_____

11. One hour ago, you were offered a free trip to a place you have wanted to travel to for quite some time. Where would you be going?

_____

_____

12. How do you feel about your size? Are you always on a diet? Or are you always waiting to lose a few pounds before going shopping? (Be truthful here! This is only for you.)

_____

_____

13. They say you can tell a lot about a

person's image by the car they choose to drive. What about you? What are you looking for in a car? If you don't have one, what would you look for?

_____

_____

14. How and where would you most like to live? Home, apartment, houseboat, tent? City, country, suburbs?

_____

_____

15. What type of work do you do? What type of work would you like to do, if you're not doing what you'd like to?

_____

_____

16. What are your criteria for a good friend? How long do you keep friends?

_____

_____

17. If you could be anywhere you wanted to be right now, where would you be and why?

_____

_____

YOUR ANSWERS

Let's go over your answers. I will tell you how I look at the answers and give you some clues as to how each question plays into determining your style. Read through all the answers. Check those that you most identify with. Then count your responses.

1. Hair Spray

The woman who is least likely to wear hair spray is either a **Sporty** or a **Romantic**.

A **Sporty** woman just doesn't want to bother. She's run the brush through and it looks fine. She's out the door. The key for her is low maintenance. I find that a Sporty woman tends not to have too much hair trauma. She'll complain that her hair is boring. What that really means is she rarely has "bad" hair days like the rest of us.

Romantics love natural looks, and to them, the fewer chemicals they have to use the better.

A **Traditional** woman will use hair spray to keep her hair looking the same all day. Sometimes her hair gets droopy by the end of the day. She'll often use Aqua Net or White Rain. She will buy what's on sale; she's not a brand hog. She also doesn't do anything too daring.

The **Classic** woman generally buys "sa-lon" spray. She often knows the name of the current hot product; not out of snobbishness, it's simply part of her demeanor. She just knows who's who in hair care, and often has the most timeless haircut of all. She'll have her hair deep conditioned routinely, out of habit. She's not compulsive about it, it's simply her "style." A Classic goes with the trends, so if it's in, she'll wear it, if not, she won't.

If she needs it, the **Dramatic** woman will use a whole bottle to achieve the look she desires. The way her hair feels does not matter to her, it's the statement she makes when she enters the room that counts. Her appearance is what matters. The brand is not always as vital here as how strong it is. If the most expensive spray won't hold her hair, she'll buy the cheapest. Her hair spray is used to achieve her "look."

A **Trendy** woman laughs at this question. She asks if I'm kidding. She buys it when she needs it and uses it when called for. If her hair is being worn loose and free this year, the spray sits on the shelf. If she's dyed it green and is wearing it spiked, she'll use a ton. She gives it no thought. She uses it only if she has to. Brand? If her friend owns the company, or the company supports her favorite charity, she'll buy it. Price is not important to her. She also doesn't linger for hours over what brand to buy.

Getting the idea? Now, let's see how you answered the rest of the questions. Make a check mark next to the style type that is most like your answer.

2. Makeup

The **Sporty** woman most often writes "I don't know." She tends to have the most eclectic makeup kit. Usually it is collected from various sources over the years. Makeup simply isn't a priority for her. My friend Susan is a typical Sporty. She resisted buying Maybelline for years until I suggested it to her. She realized that this was the perfect cosmetic company for her naturally Sporty style.

A **Romantic** woman most often comes up with Almay, Revlon, or Clinique. (Women who are allergic often say Almay or Clinique, too, and they can be of any style.) The key with a Romantic is that her makeup looks soft and is used only to enhance her natural features.

A **Traditional** woman has been using the same company for years. A name that frequently comes up on a Traditional's quiz is Estee Lauder. Overall, she tends to stick with one company.

A **Classic** woman tends to be very loyal to a company such as Lancôme or Borghese. She likes to use makeup that she can wear with everything. This is the woman who instinctively knows which shade of lipstick to wear with her various outfits and tends to have quite a bit of it. She believes in the importance of paying more for good makeup.

With a **Dramatic** woman, the brand of makeup isn't as important as the effect. Although she will go with any line as dramatic as she is, Chanel is possibly one for her.

A **Trendy** is always looking for whatever suits her current hair color. She'll wear her makeup differently when she's a blonde than when she's a brunette.

Tip: Take a look at a cosmetic company's ads. What style type are they targeting? Determining how to apply your makeup begins with finding the company that portrays an image that matches your own. You can update your look each season by getting a makeover at your favorite cosmetic counter in a department store or looking at their new ads for the coming season. Remember: *congruence*.

Tip: Most cosmetic companies are happy to send you information about their products. This is a good way to begin to create a more streamlined look to your whole package.

---

3. Haircuts

A **Sporty** woman appears to be relaxed with her hair. However, she is very concerned with the cut because low maintenance matters to her, and she knows it begins with a good cut. Luckily, Sporty women tend to have great hair. Sportys may be "laid back and natural" in other areas, but nothing freaks a Sporty woman out more than a bad haircut. She'll wear hats, sneak out the back door at work, or call in sick for a while.

The **Romantic** woman's hair can be short or long, any color. What matters to her is the feel and the movement. She wants her hair to simply be soft and feminine. Romantics often will wear bows or hair ornaments and look quite lovely. As long as the look is romantic, they won't mind. They're not going to go to a salon and get the latest style.

A **Traditional** woman has had the same haircut since high school. Yet I find that she often is the one who has had haircut nightmares. She'll get tired of her hair on Monday and in a panic book an appointment and get a "new style." A change is what she gets, often to her horror. If she asked me, I'd probably tell her that since she'll only grow it back to what it was, take some time and work on it. All of us have had bad cuts; it's the way you handle it that gives us a clue to your particular style.

A **Classic** woman will often tell you of her one haircut nightmare and laugh. She is quick to learn what works for her and stick with it. She'll only make a change after she's heard dozens of people suggest it ("You'd look great with short hair"), and she's thought about it for a year. She'll often do it gradually, too. From long hair, she'll go for bangs first, and perhaps it'll be months or even a year before she'll go to shoulder length and then short. Everything with her takes time and thought. She's not in a hurry. She's not out to make a grand statement.

Dramatic women tend to take the least risk with their haircuts. Think about Joan Collins or Liz Taylor. Lots of hair spray, but not a lot of change. When they do change, it's often well planned. Think of the gray streak Liz Taylor added to her hair—it looked sensational and dramatic, hence we all noticed. A Dramatic almost never has an "Oops . . ."

On the other hand, a **Trendy** may have an "I don't care" or "It'll grow" attitude. A Trendy hires a hairdresser and then works with him. She may decide to change the color or the length, or cut it all off or grow it long. This is an integral part of her image. She is the most current and is often slightly ahead of what's going to happen. She'll set the trend. I find Trendys tend to answer this question with, "I figure out what I want to look like this month and then do it. If it doesn't work, I'll change it."

4. Nails

The **Sporty** woman will have short, manicured nails, often with clear polish or no polish at all. More often than not, she's trying to keep up with them. She'll start a regular routine of nail care and then miss an appointment to go play tennis and her nails are shot. They seem to be always on a Sporty woman's mind, but she never quite has the time to keep them up. Just when she has them looking good, she'll get a call to play softball.

A **Romantic** woman often has short nails. If she wears polish, it's often pink. She often plays an instrument or uses her hands in a way that prevents her from having long nails.

If she does have long nails, it is to match her beautiful, soft hands.

A **Traditional** woman will have short trim nails that match her reserved life-style.

A **Classic** woman will always have a proper nail length. While Trendys or Dramatics may grow them long for effect at times, a Classic rarely would. Even if she has fake nails put on, they're always a "real" length. This is a very important part of maintenance for a Classic. You can almost always spot her by the "current" polish style. In the spring she'll often have a French manicure (if it's in style), and in the fall, red.

There is always something about a **Dramatic** woman that stands out: sometimes it's her talent, other times her eyes, or maybe simply her personality. A Dramatic woman's hands match this tendency. While she may have long acrylic nails, she can just as easily have long red nails.

Trendys don't concern themselves with nails. If they want them, they'll buy them.

5. Shoes

The **Sporty** woman is easily identified by her array of casual and flat shoes. The sneaker is her staple, and you can bet she has a few different kinds of boots in her closet. Almost always, her dressy heels seem out of place on her and they are the hardest thing for her to buy.

A **Romantic** woman's closet is made up of soft silhouettes. She's got a ton of strappy sandals and huaraches; her idea of a dressy work shoe is a slingback or open toe. Even her tennis shoes are somehow always lined with soft pink or blue. She doesn't care about the brand name, just so long as it feels good and is well made. Unlike the Traditional woman, she buys what feels good to her.

The **Traditional** woman has been buying the same brand name for years. Her mother bought it and it worked then, too. She buys moderate well-made shoes. She likes to buy leather shoes rather than man-made, and always prefers products made in her country rather than elsewhere.

She'll wear "reasonable" heel heights, but more often than not goes to work in flats and puts on a heel once she gets there. She wears sneakers to walk the dog, weed the garden, or take the kids to Little League. Unlike the Sporty woman, who will wear her shoes to death, the Traditional woman will take care of her shoes and keep them for years.

The **Classic** woman prefers to wear comfortable heels; therefore she buys only the best brand names. The Classic woman may have quite a few pairs of shoes to her name, and she's not afraid of buying man-made shoes.

If you want to see the shoe of the moment, look to see what a **Dramatic** woman is wearing on her feet. Whether it's slingbacks or platforms, if it's current, it's on her foot. She wears the latest designer names. She likes the best and that's what a label means to her. She's most likely to have quite a few heels in her closet, since she makes a more dramatic entrance in them. She generally doesn't own sneakers, and if she does, she only wears them when her trainer is at the house or she's at the gym.

Remember that a **Trendy** woman sets the trends. She doesn't care if it doesn't look right to the rest of us. If it works for her and she's comfortable, that's all that matters. Trendys don't choose to be "trendy," it comes naturally. Katharine Hepburn wore sneakers with her man-tailored trousers in the 1940s. It's highly unlikely that she was trying to make a statement; the look just worked for her. That is precisely what Trendys do. Brand names? She doesn't even notice. If it works, it's on her foot.

6. Panty Hose

A **Sporty** woman is lost in the field of panty hose. She deems it a necessary evil. She'll wear the right color but secretly wonders if other women rip up as many pairs of panty hose as often as she does. She buys what seems right but wonders if she can get away without any, and sometimes does.

A **Romantic** woman wears panty hose when it is appropriate. She doesn't give it too much thought. If she does know the brand she buys, it's because it feels good. It's simply not that important to her.

A **Traditional** woman buys her hose at supermarkets, and she'll often buy the least expensive pair that will get the job done. Color variety isn't her concern; she'll wear hose to match her skin tone or skirt. Color would be a splurge, but often only for a special dress, not for everyday. She rarely runs out, but since she goes through lots of them, she may buy in bulk.

A **Classic** woman will buy her panty hose in bulk, sometimes through the mail (often at outlet stores). She likes to match her hose and her skirt and shoes, opting for black or navy or white. If a nude leg is "in" that season, she may wear it, too.

A **Dramatic** woman always says yes to panty hose. She owns every conceivable style and wears them all. She often has a good sense of color matching and isn't afraid to wear a daring pattern of hose.

A **Trendy** woman once looked at me and said, "I don't know if I still have any." If it fits into her look of the moment, she'll be well stocked. If not, she might not be. Name brands? She's not afraid of them, but she doesn't shop for them either. She isn't price conscious, spending more than it's worth if panty hose make the outfit.

7. Undergarments

a) Shoulder pads?

Sportys don't understand why anyone needs them; they certainly don't.

Romantics don't really notice if their clothes don't have them.

Traditional women often rip them out, not caring for them.

Classics pour them on; they like looking proportional.

Dramatics can't live without them.

Trendys can take or leave them.

b and c) Bras and panties

Sporty women buy good, strong underwear. Unlike a Classic or Dramatic, who will wear sexy underwear for themselves, Sportys need a reason for wearing something other than the plain old clean pair that Mom told them to never leave the house without.

Romantic women like soft colors and floral designs. They don't always buy expensive underwear, but they buy very soft, natural items.

Traditional women typically wear traditional underwear. They often buy good quality underwear on sale.

Classic: don't let her fool you. She's got on some sexy underwear. And she likes to spend money on it.

To a **Dramatic,** underwear must be as dramatic as they are—they love bustiers.

Trendys ooze sexuality and can wear plain cotton or lace, whatever suits them at the moment.

d) Slips

A **Sporty** woman wears a slip as a basic necessity. She thinks that she's supposed to wear them under dresses or skirts, so she may wear one even if she doesn't need to—just to be sure.

A **Romantic** woman rarely has a use for a slip. The type of clothes she wears don't call for slips very often, so she doesn't have them. She probably has a few that were from her mother or grandmother. However, she'll have leggings or bloomers to wear under a sheer skirt.

Traditional women have at least two: a half-slip and a full-length slip.

A **Classic** woman will almost always have the basics, one black, one white, and one beige slip.

Dramatics will often have them in assorted colors.

Trendys? A Trendy once told me, "I just bought an antique slip. It looks like a dress so I'll wear it as one." She did.

e) Nightgowns

Sporty women sometimes have something frilly or silky. But more often than not, they have a favorite oversized T-shirt with a team insignia on it.

Romantic women will have frilly lace and floral-patterned sleepwear, and almost always cotton. If it's sexy, it's silk or satin.

Traditional women always have nightgowns. They wear their flannels in the winter and their cottons in the summer.

Classic women often have nice classic

styles, including some not-so-classic teddy sets to wear to bed.

Dramatic women only wear their nightgowns for effect. They are likely to have an entire ensemble to dazzle any viewer.

A **Trendy** once answered this question with: "You mean negligee?" They don't often wear nightgowns, but if they do they don't care if the whole world knows it's an old Donald Duck T-shirt.

8. Designers

Designers' names usually give me a good indication of style type. If a client doesn't have a designer listed, I ask her whose styles best represent what is in her present wardrobe. They usually fall into one of these categories.

Sporty—Esprit, Gap, Guess, Lizwear.

Romantic—Laura Ashley, Carole Little, Karen Kane.

Traditional—J. G. Hook, Jones New York, Leslie Faye, Anne Klein.

Classics—Adrienne Vittadini, JH Collectibles, Elizabeth, Ellen Tracy.

Dramatics—Norma Kamali, Bob Mackie, Escada, Tahari, Armani.

Trendys—DKNY, Betsey Johnson, Andrea Jovine (but they often have dozens of original pieces).

9. Exercise

We're in **Sporty**s element here. She loves to do natural things like a Romantic, she

has nothing against weights, and you'll often find her in the weight room at the local gym with the men. She's frequently into several sports.

Romantics tend to horseback ride or do things that are nature-oriented, sometimes doing things that would surprise you. One client I worked with was a Romantic and she loved to go white-water rafting in some pretty treacherous waters!

When I travel the country doing seminars, I frequently see quite a few **Traditional** women walking the local mall in the morning for exercise. Their sport is golf or sometimes tennis. You won't find many Traditional women playing racquetball, but along with their Sporty sisters, you may find them on the high seas sailing.

A **Classic** will never go too far overboard to exercise, although she will pass up other offers in order to stick to a regular routine. No matter what, it is unlikely that she would give up her sweets. If she does get on a boat, she'll prefer a motorboat—less work that way.

Dramatics often exercise with a trainer at home or using a tape. Although they may horseback ride, they are more likely to be at the races on opening day in the latest outfit, rather than actually riding a horse.

Trendys exercise to challenge themselves. They're the ones who workout furiously when they've had enough of being out of shape. It becomes their newest craze. They don't care how they look and often they're wearing their brother's old gym clothes. Look to a Trendy to try anything at least once and not care what anyone else has to say.

10. Passion
Although there is a broad range of ways to answer this, there are certain things that I look for.

Sportys are the first to walk for AIDS or run for freedom. Their involvement is almost always physical in some way. Sportys are healthy and will do anything to promote it.

Romantics are usually passionate about environmental issues. They'll lick envelopes for Save the Whales or volunteer to man the phones for the Sierra Club.

A **Traditional's** passion is in relation to her children or family; she'll pledge money for the local educational channel.

Classics are passionate about some cause in relation to their work or community. They'll protest by writing letters or making calls; while you may see them on the picket line, you generally won't see them organizing it.

Dramatics will either say they are most passionate about their career or a cause relating to human beings in some way.

Trendys will tend to express their personal spiritual "beliefs" or current philosophy—through their own choice of expression.

11. Free Trip
A **Sporty** woman has the hardest time with this question. She'd love to go whitewater rafting or scuba diving or sky diving or . . . Bet on her to pick something where she's going to be quite active.

A **Romantic** woman will choose a place of great natural beauty. She may choose to travel to a famous city—maybe to live in an artist's apartment and borrow their passionate life for a month. Or she may choose to visit an island to ride horses or run along deserted beaches and collect shells.

A **Traditional** woman often chooses travel to a city where she can visit a person she knows. It doesn't matter where. She isn't always comfortable away from home, so she likes an anchor in a new place.

A **Classic** woman frequently travels for a living, so the idea of traveling and sightseeing isn't always appealing to her. She opts for a fun "package" type of vacation, like a Club Med or a spa. Or she may go somewhere to just lie on a beach and read.

A **Dramatic** would love to go somewhere to be seen. Monaco, Paris, shopping in Italy, a cruise to Europe.

A **Trendy** would go wherever she was in the mood to go. An African safari, rafting down the Amazon, or a trip to see her mom in Detroit—it wouldn't matter to her, since she goes by whatever she feels like doing at that moment.

12. Your Dieting Status

What makes a **Sporty** different from a Romantic here? Well, she's going to look for foods to increase her endurance and lower her fat intake. While other women will eat this way sporadically, for a Sporty woman, it's a way of life. A Sporty woman will even go for low-fat desserts and stick with it!

A **Romantic** woman likes to eat healthy foods. She is sometimes a vegetarian (this is not to be confused with a Trendy, who takes on being a vegetarian as a "cause" and who may eat nothing that was killed in any violent way). If she eats poultry, it'll be organic. Diet? The only diet she's on is a healthy one.

A **Traditional** woman is often on a "diet" of some kind. Or she'll say she's "watching what she eats."

That's different from the **Classic**, who says she likes to "watch what I eat." The Classic will eat when she is hungry and sometimes crams down some junk food if she's in a rush.

A **Dramatic** will often use her "diet" as an excuse for eating or not eating something. Whether or not she actually is dieting is another matter. I think it must have been a Dramatic who coined the phrase "One can never be too rich or too thin."

A **Trendy** will always tell the truth here, if asked. She doesn't try to hide anything: it's not in her nature. If she's on a mission to slim down, she'll just avoid dessert. Or she'll eat anything she chooses and not feel the need to make any excuses.

13. What do you look for in buying a car?

At this point you are beginning to get a good sense of each of the different style types. They may all choose to drive the same car, but each will have a different rationale.

Let's say all our women choose a Honda.

A **Sporty** will want her car to run well; she doesn't have the time to wait around for repairs!

A **Romantic** may want a fuel-efficient car that runs well so that the ozone layer isn't ruined as fast.

A **Traditional** will want a car that is good value.

A **Classic** wants something that never goes out of style.

A **Dramatic** would choose a car based on her need for creature comforts.

A **Trendy** may feel that she wants something that will go with all her "looks." A Honda? Sure, if it's a motorcycle.

14. Where do you live?

A **Sporty** is going to live near her favorite activities.

A **Romantic** ideally would choose a home in the woods. However, more often than not it's her bedroom that tells her tale. She'll have floral and lace pillows everywhere.

A **Traditional** woman is most apt to be found in a suburban home or an apartment complex.

A **Classic** will live in a nice home or apartment. She often chooses to live in a lovely neighborhood whether or not she can afford it, since she likes an upscale environment.

A **Dramatic** woman would choose to live in opulence. Wherever she may reside, it must look and feel very rich and lavish—unless it's a dramatically poor loft.

A **Trendy** woman can be found in a loft, a renovated warehouse, or a houseboat. It doesn't really matter to the Trendy woman, and although she's more apt to be found in a neighborhood of artists instead of suburbia, she could move into a retirement village to "get away from it all." Expect the unexpected from her.

15. Your Career?

A **Sporty** can show up anywhere. She may be an attorney, a horse breeder, or a chef. Remember that she likes exercise, so she can also be found as a personal trainer or an aerobics instructor. Many Sportys are models or actresses—their fresh wholesome appearance makes them appealing to the public.

A **Romantic** is often an artist of some kind. She may be a healer or a musician, or even own her own store. Romantics are the least likely to be found in the corporate world,

though if they are, they are loyal, caring, and thorough employees.

A **Traditional** woman frequently chooses a low-profile position. She is not interested in climbing the corporate ladder, and as a result you may find her in a travel agency, as an office worker, or somewhere near home. Since she often has children, she likes to be close to them, so work is seldom the most important thing to her.

A **Classic** woman is often on her way up the ladder. Corporate or not, she is the perfect businesswoman. She could easily be self-employed, for she has drive, motivation, and direction.

A **Dramatic** will definitely have a high-visibility position. Whether she owns a company or is an actress, she's chosen a career based upon status and visibility. Public relations, theater, or fashion are just a few areas where you'll spot her. But don't rule out an office job for her. The important thing to remember is that Ms. D is really the one running the show.

A **Trendy** can be found anywhere! She can make doughnuts, manage musical bands, or be a hairdresser. The key with a Trendy is that no matter where she is, she'll be doing her own thing. You won't often find her in the corporate world, but if you do, she's in consulting or owns the company. Trendys do not make good employees: they are too independent and often go their own way. They do, however, make excellent salespeople, since they can easily reach out to many different types of people.

16. Friendship

I find that most women have good friends, and that they've had them for a long time. Here is what I have heard each style type say to me about their friendships.

Sporty—While she may have close ties from her childhood, she is often closest to those with whom she pursues her favorite sports and activities.

Romantic—Like her Traditional sister, she'll often maintain friendships from childhood.

Traditional—She still has friends from second grade! She never loses track of people and always remembers birthdays and holidays. While she may not be as flamboyant as a Trendy or Dramatic, she quite often has a full social calendar.

Classic—Since a Classic woman's focus is often her work, that is where her social contacts often lie. She will have outside friends, but she often has a hard time seeing them because of her work commitments. A Classic also easily forgets birthdays and anniversaries.

Dramatic—As long as she is the center of attention, she can maintain friends for life. She is a true friend, but she would never pick someone to be friends with who might outshine her.

Trendy—She is friends with everyone. She doesn't care about another's social standing or what they do or how much money they make. She treats everyone the same open way.

17. If you could be anywhere you want to be, right now, where would you be and why?

Sporty—Playing her favorite sport.

Romantic—In her favorite garden having tea.

Traditional—With her kids, husband, or significant other.

Classic—Getting a raise, or making a deal.

Dramatic—Anywhere but here.

Trendy—Right where she is.

Take stock of your answers. Whatever style type dominates is your style type. If you have a second style that comes on strong, then that is probably your accent style. *Be careful not to let your accent style dominate in your wardrobe.*

Are you between two different types? Consider these tiebreakers:

Romantics and Sportys are closely linked and often the easiest to mistake. While Sportys will wear spandex and exercise gear, anything that represents movement, Romantics won't want to wear anything too clingy, preferring long flowing fabrics.

Classics and Traditionals are closely linked. The difference is that a Classic is more designer conscious. She'll buy expensive designer looks, while her Traditional sister won't mind a nondesigner suit. A Traditional would rather have real pearls, while her Classic sister will opt for large Anne Klein II jewelry that adds a bold statement to her classic lines.

Trendys and Dramatics are closely linked. They differ in that Dramatics often do what they do to make a statement, while Trendys don't really care what you may think. Dramatics don't care what the fabric is, as long as it looks sensational, and they will endure far more fashion pain than any other style type. A Trendy, on the other hand, will only wear what she likes and what makes her feel good. She is not oblivious to style, she just doesn't care to vie for attention. If she gets it, fine; if not, who cares?

THE SECOND STEP

Buy a few magazines and tear out pictures that appeal to you. Place them in three piles:

1. The first pile should contain pictures that are "you."

2. The next pile is for everything that definitely is not you, will never be you, could never be you.
3. Finally, create a third pile of pictures of who you'd like to be.

Using the pictures from piles one and three—who you are and who you want to be—make a collage. Go get a piece of posterboard and some glue. Some women have cut out additional pictures and made collages with images having nothing to do with fashion. That works, too. I find that putting together a collage helps individualize your elements of style. However your collage turns out, it is part of the road map to unlocking your personal style.

Study your collage as if someone else made it. The key to interpreting your collage is to look at what the woman who made it is trying to tell you.

Are there looks on this collage that do not match the woman's life-style? Do they all match?

Is anything on it in her wardrobe already?

Or is there nothing that she presently wears?

Is it mostly who she is or who she'd like to be?

These are the questions I consider when I'm interpreting a collage. Sometimes the inconsistencies are as important as the consistencies.

In short, I'm looking for congruence, or lack of it. I'm trying to find ways to make my client more congruent.

It's rare that a collage doesn't tell the whole story, but in that rare case, I have my clients do a statement. A statement can help to pick up additional clues and piece together the full story about a person.

THE THIRD STEP

Write a statement. For example, a client once had a collage covered with elegant pictures, but her statement said that she was ready to live a quiet life in the country.

We had to bridge the gap between these two ideas and find out which one was real, or this woman would always be chasing two different lives. Writing your statement is simple:

Outline the focus of your life and what you'd like your wardrobe to be for you. This helps to make you see any conflicts you may have that are preventing you from having a functioning wardrobe.

Writing a statement about yourself will give you the objectivity of a fashion expert.

When you read it, try to do so without judgment. What does is it tell you about the woman who wrote it?

Chapter Three

THE STYLE WHEEL

The style wheel is a visual guide to each of the six styles. Although each style is covered in depth in its own chapter, the wheel will give you an idea of where you fit in relation to the other style types. Let's take a spin around beginning with Sporty.

The **Sporty** woman is all about play. She is in the first position on the wheel, and the elements of her personality (while uniquely her own), do blend Trendy and Romantic. Since she is before Romantic, she sometimes wishes she could dress more like a Romantic. Why? It is the nature of the circle to admire the type after you.

Second on the wheel is **Romantic**. She gains her love of the outdoors from Sporty, although she isn't quite as active as her predecessor. And, she learns respect for family values from her Traditional sister, whom *she*

precedes. Unlike Ms. Traditional, she isn't above wrecking a home in the name of love. Her key word is *love* because it is the thing that matters to her above all else.

The first stop on the upper hemisphere of the wheel is **Traditional**. The Traditional woman has high regard for her family and tends to be less of a career woman than her Classic sister above. She may have a thriving career, but what she deeply values is tradition. Her clothing does not hold the same importance as it does for a Classic. She is also not willing to throw everything to the wind for love like a Romantic. She is the blend of what has come before and what lies ahead.

In the fourth position on the wheel is **Classic**. She is the typical career woman. Her career dictates her values, and while family is important to her, she knows they will under-

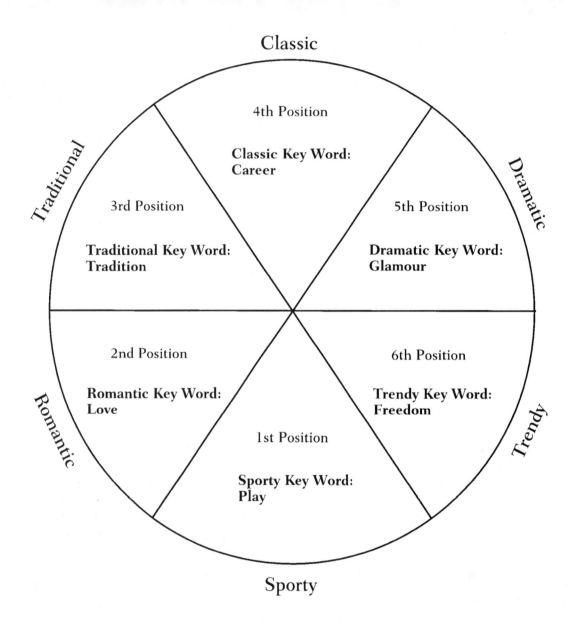

Classic

Traditional

Dramatic

4th Position

**Classic Key Word:
Career**

3rd Position

5th Position

**Traditional Key Word:
Tradition**

**Dramatic Key Word:
Glamour**

2nd Position

6th Position

**Romantic Key Word:
Love**

**Trendy Key Word:
Freedom**

1st Position

Romantic

Trendy

**Sporty Key Word:
Play**

Sporty

stand (hopefully). Since she is right behind Dramatic, it is the glamorous woman that she greatly admires. On some level, she deeply wishes she could be more dramatic. Ms. Classic maintains a blend of tradition and drama in her personality.

Nestled between Classic and Trendy is **Dramatic.** Her key word is *glamour.* Graced with a natural presence, she is one step short of the daring Trendy and secretly wonders if Trendy is really as nonchalant as she appears.

She is. Nonchalant, that is. **Trendy** is the woman who will laugh when faced with what others would consider scandal. She may appear uncaring about some things at times, but that's not necessarily true. She simply does not get ruffled about scandal the way her Dramatic friends would. While she does envy Sporty's natural athletic ability, there is nothing Ms. Trendy can't do if she sets her mind to it. She is a self-starter from the word go.

ABOVE AND BELOW THE EQUATOR

The line that runs horizontally through the wheel splits the style types into upper and lower quadrants. Those in the upper hemisphere—Traditional, Classic, and Dramatic—are outer-directed types. They care more about what others think of them than they'll often admit. The Traditional woman is eager to please those she loves, the Classic wishes to excel in her career, and the Dramatic wants to make a statement every time she enters a room. These types rely upon others' opinions more than they'd care to admit.

While the Traditional woman may not be a designer label show off, she does enjoy clothing. Classic is much more daring than her Traditional sister, willing to take risks with her looks to impress others with her taste. Interestingly, Dramatic's need for attention is often inbred. She is not necessarily a deliberate scene stealer, she just naturally draws attention. This ability to draw crowds becomes comfortable over time and she comes to expect it.

The outer world, and other people, play heavily into the sphere of the upper hemisphere.

Each of the Style types residing below the equator is inner-directed. Trendy, Sporty, and Romantic are all in tune with their feelings. The temperature inside is far more important to them than the temperature outside.

Trendy has to do what she *believes* to be right. Sporty must first be in tune with her body and the earth before she can relate to others. For Romantic, being in touch with her feelings is what drives her. These types tend to be in touch with themselves.

It's not that any of the upper types aren't in touch with themselves, but being so self-aware simply isn't as important to them as to the types below the equator.

Now that you know a little about you, let's see how your style relates to that of your neighbors.

FACTS ABOUT THE WHEEL

Let's consider where you are on the wheel. Who's before you? After you? There tends to be a natural friction with the style type after you, since they may intimidate you. It is in our nature to want to be more like those whose styles we admire, and the wheel is no exception. Each style type secretly covets the good qualities of the style type after them. Let's go around the wheel and see how we relate to the style type after us.

Sporty is fun, free, and outgoing. Her natural demeanor is refreshing. There are times when she may wish she were more of a Romantic.

Key mistake: Trying to wear Romantic outfits. They never quite feel good on her.

Romantic is as caring as can be. But there are times when she wishes that she could be more traditional and not so ruled by her emotional state.

Key mistake: Trying to live her life in a traditional style. She will never feel good about her life unless she is immersed in love.

Traditional is a very concerned friend. She is the lady to confide in when you need someone to talk to. There are times, however, when she longs for the polish of her Classic sister.

Key mistake: Trying to wear classic styles and adding traditional accents. It gives the appearance of someone who is dressing to impress.

Classic is controlled, disciplined, and energetic. She is very passionate about her work and is driven to be the best. She is easily intimidated by Dramatic's flashiness and sometimes wishes she were more flamboyant.

Key mistake: Trying to wear dramatic outfits as classics. While she can carry off some bolder silhouettes, she can look hopelessly overdone and create the exact opposite of the impression she is vying for.

Dramatic is flamboyant and in control. She is almost always center of attention, and there are very few times when she is not. She wishes she could adopt Trendy's nonchalance.

Key mistake: Trying to adopt the ease of a Trendy. This only makes her appear sloppy.

Trendy takes the boldness of a Dramatic and mixes it with her own brand of free-spiritedness and winds up being quite polished, even when she is "slumming." She doesn't, however, have Sporty's finesse with workout gear and hence her casual wear can sometimes be downright sloppy. Lucky for her, she doesn't care.

Key mistake: Even if there were one to make, Trendy wouldn't care, so why name one.

The style type before you may feel like a baby sister who is tagging along all the time. Hers is the style you may look down upon as being not quite up to your standards. They may have some fabulous qualities, but they are hard to see because they annoy us. But, without a style type preceding you, there would be no one to pick on!

Keep this in mind: The style type that precedes you has much to teach you. From her, you often learn good habits. Don't just think that because you are past her you are better than her. It is the type before you who has the patience to learn that which you may snub as inconsequential.

For example:

Sporty may look down at Trendy's doing anything she wants. When in reality, Sporty could learn much from Trendy in terms of flexibility.

Romantic may dismiss Sporty's athletic ability, but much of her personal problems may stem from lack of exercise.

Traditional may not respect Romantic's living her life governed by love, but Traditional could be reminded at times how important love is in the family equation. She may push her loved ones too hard from time to time.

Classic could learn to be more thoughtful of others from Traditional, who never forgets birthdays or anniversaries and always remembers those she loves. Classic can be callous at times.

Dramatic can learn much from Classic, whose passionate dedication to hard work is at times awe inspiring. While Dramatics love praise, it is their Classic sister who is not afraid of earning it.

Trendy will learn about behaving in a more distinguished manner from her Dramatic sister, who is the style expert when it comes to protocol.

It's important to realize that each style type is valuable and wonderful in its own way.

If you dress in the previous style, it can make you appear dowdy and drag you down.

Opposites

By now you are beginning to get a picture of how you relate to a few of the other style types. But which style will complement you the most?

The style directly opposite you tends to be the most complementary. When it comes to what is missing from your wardrobe, it is often the life-style opposite you. Interestingly, that is the style that we can borrow ideas from to add to our wardrobe.

What do I mean by that?

There is no competition between opposites. They are so diametrically opposed, there is no way that one could mistake the other. The other thing to consider is that each needs the other for balance.

Let's take a look at the **Sporty/Classic** dynamic first.

Sporty often craves a more classic look. She is never quite able to achieve it, though, because it isn't her. However, Sporty can borrow a few elements of a Classic's style and look quite elegant. It's easy for them to both wear knits. Sporty can wear a knit two-piece ensemble or a knit dress easily. Even if they have Classic lines, they can work beautifully on her.

Classic, on the other hand, has problems finding relaxed, casual looks for herself. She is always polished. Therefore, Sporty's relaxed styling can be helpful to Ms. Classic. She can pull a few pieces from Sporty and make them her own.

Romantics and **Dramatics**, too, have an interesting dynamic. The most flowing and elegant romantic gowns can look sensational on Ms. Dramatic.

While Dramatic desires to be center stage, Romantic wants to be appreciated. These two can be quite compatible, often sharing accessories such as a cuff bracelet, which is decidedly Romantic, but a sensational companion to a Dramatic's boldness.

Traditional/Trendy. Two style types could not seem more opposite, yet be more similar. Trendy often borrows from Ms. Traditional's wardrobe choices and does wild things to her accessories or funks them out.

Ms. Traditional can be so stark and simple that, at times, she is more trendy than the current trends dictate.

If you must borrow something, do it from the style type on the opposite side of the wheel. But only a little; if you go overboard, you'll look out of place.

Opposite style types often hold opposite characteristics. For example:

A Sporty is fun and free while a Classic is controlled and disciplined.

A Romantic is all about love and feelings and a Dramatic is very sexy and bold.

Traditionals believe in family values while Trendys treasure their own values.

A WORD ABOUT ACCENT TYPES

Now that you understand the wheel and your placement on it, you can probably spot your accent type.

Accent types can change over time. When Sporty looks were all the rage in the 1980s, everyone wore bike shorts and stirrup pants. Even Elizabeth Taylor, a true Dramatic, rode motorcycles with her friend Malcolm Forbes.

When romantic looks came in, we all entertained touches of romance. But only a Romantic should buy like crazy.

We all play with different types, but always remember that the focus of whatever you are wearing should always be your primary style type.

A FINAL THOUGHT ON THE WHEEL

There was a time when each of the styles created waves. Different eras dictate who the current "rebels" are.

Although Trendy is the most independent of styles, there was a time when being a Classic was shocking. A woman with a career? Heavens.

A Sporty child in New York City might stand out, while if she lived on a farm she would blend in. Each of the styles fit well in some places and stand out in others.

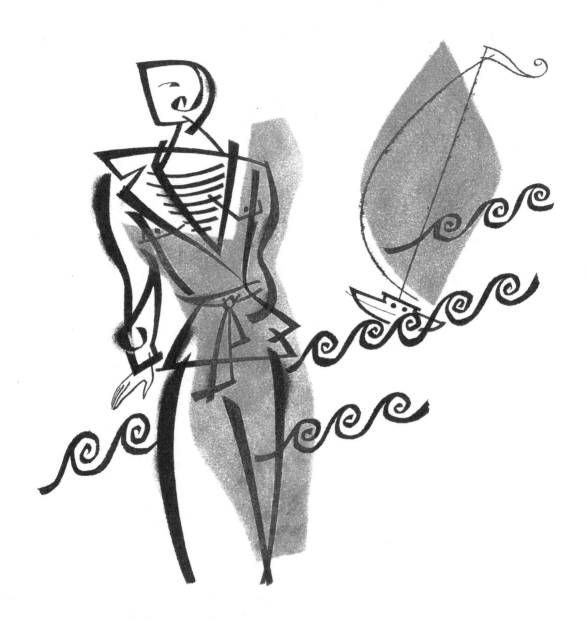

Chapter Four

SPORTY

The word *natural* crops up quite a bit where Sporty's concerned, because there is a natural ease to this woman's demeanor. Her appeal is also attributed to Sporty's naïveté. She is unpretentious. Period. This is not a woman who needs to put others down to build herself up. Not much for gossip, Sporty shies away from it. This woman is genuine and fun.

The Sporty woman is naturally body conscious. She's keenly aware of her body as a machine, and food is the fuel that keeps her going. She is the woman who eats right, exercises, and takes her vitamins. To her, the clothes have nothing to decorate if she isn't healthy and in great shape.

Hers is the wardrobe that is versatile, as well it has to be, and she may change a few times a day. These clothes have to be functional, and that is the number-one consideration when she dresses. Although she can dress very elegantly, her closet probably has more athletic shoes than high heels.

Her home is comfortable, and although she rarely formally entertains, her door is always open to people dropping by. While Ms. Sporty may have a high-profile career, she still maintains the ultimate casual life-style and things rarely, if ever, ruffle her feathers. You won't find her sitting behind a desk; she's always on the go. Most Sportys find careers where they can maintain constant movement. They need the activity to keep them from feeling sedentary.

Sportys by nature are enthusiastic and fun people. They are often involved in activities with their mates that would normally be reserved for "boys." They are the first to hop on a motorcycle or learn mountain climbing.

Her interests include the daring and extreme. Sporty fashion models always seem to be the most popular—Cheryl Tiegs in the '70s and Christie Brinkley in the 1980s. Why? Sportys have an air of availability about them.

No matter where on the social scale a Sporty comes from, she tends to be very gracious and accepting of others. A Sporty draws from the idea of sportsmanship—if you want to play, join in. It didn't require an invitation on the playground, and to a Sporty, life doesn't either.

Sporty, however, may be out of sorts when it comes to dressing for an occasion where clothing is not dictated by the day's particular needs. Swimming requires a suit, golf a golf outfit, skiing . . . well, ski clothes. Ms. Sporty's biggest problem is what to wear when the clothes aren't clearly defined, like a "casual" sit-down dinner at the boss's home.

Esprit is one brand of clothes that's well suited to the fun and comfort this woman expects from her wardrobe.

RECOGNIZING A SPORTY

In *Pretty Woman,* Julia Roberts becomes an elegant young woman. Fortunately, she never quite loses her sporty edge, which is definitely her natural charm.

In the movie, two outfits stand out. One is the brown polka-dot dress she wears in the polo sequence. A sporty silhouette!

The other is that unforgettable red evening gown she wears to the opera. The elegance and grace Julia Roberts brings to the dress are clear, but what is important to point out is that the dress itself is sporty as well.

Why? Okay, try to imagine Elizabeth Taylor, a Dramatic, in that same red dress. It would be far too much. Red is the color of a Sporty, energetic and alive. This dress was the perfect choice for a Sporty woman like Julia Roberts.

Think too of hair, nails, and makeup. For a sporty everything is natural and easy. Nothing is too overdone.

What are the elements that make an outfit sporty?

The most important element of Sporty's clothing is that it functions as a part of her. Bear in mind that any detailing should be functional. In addition, her outfits should have a lived-in feel to them.

No one style wears T-shirts as important wardrobe elements like Sporty does. Whether a lightweight knit sweater, V neck, or her boyfriend's Hanes undershirt, this lady knows how to make lived-in both sexy and elegant.

A Sporty would not really wear a catsuit; it is not functional enough for her. However, anything in the closet that is loved and borders on another style type can be turned into a Sporty. Just make sure that the eye-catching detail or focal point is sporty.

One more important thing to remember about Sporty is her placement on the wheel. While she is in the first position, she follows Trendy. You will often see some elements that could be seen as trendy. To spot a Sporty though, always look for that lived-in feel. While any style can wear a sweatshirt, it is Sporty who wears wrinkled and torn naturally. There is a particularly femininity in a Sporty woman wearing men's clothing. Hiking shoes and boxer shorts are two examples.

> **Tip:** A popular trend happens when a look is versatile enough that it can be worn by several style types. This is why certain trends come in and gain popularity.

A SPORTY STORY

Each style type has characteristics that are shared by most women of that type. I'll use one Sporty client as an example, and show you how I gather information from a client. This should be helpful in doing it for yourself.

I first met Maya at an elegant gallery opening at a friend's home. Several times during the evening we found ourselves in the same group talking, yet we didn't speak directly to one another. I kept feeling that she had something to say to me, and I later found out that she did.

The host finally officially introduced us, saying, "Psychic, meet the fashion expert." He walked away, leaving us alone, and she said, "You will write a book about your methods." At the time, the last thing I wanted to do was write another book!

She was wearing a yellow sequined gown that was gorgeous, but too elegant for her. When she telephoned me days later and said she was told to hire me, I thought she'd heard a voice, but actually, her mother was buying my services as a gift.

Maya hailed from a very wealthy family and they had no understanding of her "work." But they did understand style, and it disturbed them that their daughter didn't. Her mother had been trying for years to get Maya interested in fashion, and when Maya expressed interest in what I did, her mother jumped at the chance.

Maya, on the other hand, had only agreed to this because she had sensed the night we met that my work was "important" in some way, although she didn't quite know how.

When I arrived at their home, the butler had me wait in the drawing room. The mansion resembled a museum, and it appeared to have been decorated by a Classic. Maya appeared soon after wearing a pair of jeans and a classic-style blouse that wasn't her.

Taking the quiz, we discovered that she was a Sporty. I told her that the next parts of the personal inventory were going to have to take place at her home. She was surprised that I knew she didn't live there. But it wasn't hard to see that her clothes wore her. She was a Sporty who had been broken. I correctly assumed her mother was the Classic in her life. And I knew that being here was not going to lend me further insight into my new client.

We arranged our next meeting at her apartment. She lived in a walk-up apartment in the city. The moment I walked in the door, I knew it was her place because it was more relaxed and sporty.

CLOSET OR COLLAGE?

I usually have my clients do the collage and statement first, but in Maya's case I felt it best to go through her closet first. I had to make sure that she would be able to spot her style before making up a collage. Her mother bought most of her clothes and I felt her collage would look more classic than sporty. My concern was that Maya would not be able to recognize her own sporty style since her mother had long ago overruled her taste.

We worked on her closet, arranging it in color order. As we worked, she began to see what was her mother's style, what was hers, and what were things that had looked good on friends, but were not her style. The Sporty slowly began to emerge. She commented that it was interesting that the sporty clothes were the pieces she wore the most and they felt more free to her.

Once we weeded out what wasn't her, I left her to do her collage and statement. Maya's collage and statement both revealed that she enjoyed city life; all the energy and people excited her. It was easy to see that she was going for a casual look, based upon the pictures. Her catsuit had been the final hold-out in her wardrobe, and when she saw that it simply didn't work, she tossed it. She also never wore it, so it wasn't as if she was throwing away something she loved. I never would have let her do that.

Her statement was very simple. She loved being in a city with such high energy and felt the most connected there. She was happy right where she was. But she wanted to feel more coordinated and not so underdressed all the time.

I had to assure her that being a Sporty didn't mean casual necessarily. It meant that she was wholesome and healthy. Her attitude toward life was basically optimistic and her energy level was high. She could look sophisticated and very sharp as a Sporty, she just needed to do this with sporty silhouettes.

Our next step was to work on her personal colors as well as adding to her now-depleted closet.

COLORS IN HER CLOSET

There were three large categories of color hanging in her closet: kelly green, royal blue, and burgundy. Of these colors, I asked her to tell me which she felt the most relaxed in. Kelly green was her reply.

The second color I wanted to know about was which one she received the most compliments on. Burgundy.

The final question I had was which color did she derive the most power from?

Royal blue.

These were what Maya's personal colors were:

1. Kelly green for who she really is,
2. Burgundy for how the world sees her, and
3. Royal blue for her power color.

All three of these colors, interestingly, are on the "winter" chart.

At the end of this chapter is a mini color glossary. This will give you a general idea of how *you* wear color.

However, I suggest you refer to the main glossary (Chapter Fourteen) for deeper insight into your choice of color. Before you read the color bio I compiled for my client, Maya, take a moment to look up the colors in the glossary and see what you come up with.

Since kelly green is how she sees herself, she is very, very open and available to others, and the burgundy tells me that others trust her intuition. The royal blue tells me that she is very confident in herself and her abilities.

It wasn't hard to see that while all three colors are on the same chart, it was not necessary for Maya to combine them, since each is powerful enough. Maya's colors were easy to build out from, because burgundy works with the deeper neutral tones of brown, black, navy, and gray; while royal works well into the deep brown and black family. And finally, kelly green is a great color to wear with her casual and outfits.

> **Tip:** The important thing to remember when building your wardrobe is to always continue to build. Never buy into a dead end. Don't buy a color that goes with nothing in your closet, or you may have made a costly mistake. Chances are you already own many of the colors that are right for you. Buying a "wrong" color can cause you to buy other "wrong" colors to go with your mistake.

THE SHOPPING LIST

How will this color information help you build a wardrobe? Look at all you know about Maya. You know who she is, what style she is, and by her colors you can tell what is deeply important to her.

All I needed to know about Maya was how she spent the bulk of her time. She worked at home, and most of her wardrobe had to be comfortable and functional. Sporty all the way. She had even chosen a profession (although she claimed it chose her) where her life-style matched her style, the best kind. Be-cause she really was starting from scratch, we made a list of all the things in her collage. This is what we came up with:

1. Colorful jeans
2. Silks, tops, and blouses
3. Funky surplus outfit, which included a hat, gloves, army pants, boots, and a pocket watch
4. A new ski outfit
5. Two "daily" dresses (for warm weather), one floral, one long linen
6. Two old plaid shirts
7. Two turtlenecks
8. Suspenders
9. A leather knapsack (instead of a purse)
10. An old sports jersey
11. A new hiking outfit.

Sporty, unlike any other style type, will wear things to shreds. I had to coerce Maya into parting with a few things only worthy of becoming cleaning rags. Next, we went into her closet and crossed the things off the "collage" list that she either already owned or could improvise.

> **Tip:** A Sporty can easily take her cue from Romantic for some dresses if need be, just be careful to make sure they have a practical element about them; ie, pockets.

We also added a few things that I knew Maya would need since these are the things most often missing from a Sporty's wardrobe:

An evening gown
A cocktail dress
A day dress (for a wedding or tea party, also functional on a cruise)
A pair of dressy slacks in any of her colors (this was to become an outfit, so we had to make sure that there was a top or jacket to go with it)

This is where Maya had to go to work on her own. I instructed her to be on the lookout for things on her list in magazines or catalogs.

> **Tip:** Make sure that any items you need for special occasions are bought in one of your three personal colors. This guarantees that your new purchases will go with the shoes and accessories you already own.

RESULTS

It took some time, but here's what Maya came up with.

1. Her day dress was found in a boutique. It had a floral design in navy and burgundy and worked beautifully with her navy sandals for more casual affairs and navy pumps for dressier.

2. The evening gown was more of a challenge. She found a cut she loved in a bridal magazine. It was a wedding dress. I suggested a seamstress, and Maya bought a cotton-blend fabric in royal blue. After modifying the original picture slightly, she had a dress made that was so stunning, I almost bought one too (until I remembered it wasn't my style). Cutting through a local department store one day, she spotted a pair of shoes in royal blue that matched perfectly.

> **Tip:** Nothing looks more horrible than a shoe that is even slightly off when you are trying to match. Don't wear shoes that are the wrong color. When in doubt, go for a neutral rather than risk mismatching.

3. In a thrift store, Maya spotted a chiffon dress in icy pink. She bought it for ten dollars and brought it to me. With its spaghetti straps, it looked like a night gown. One look at the label inside told me I was right. But, the cut and shape were perfect for Maya. She only needed something on top, a crocheted shawl or jacket. The answer came from Maya's closet. She owned a sheer white cropped top.

An old strand of pearls and white pumps were the rest of this solution.

4. Maya preferred her slacks in cotton. She traveled with her mother into warm climates, and she wanted something comfortable and easy. I suggested some wide-leg cotton pants in icy blue, with a matching floral jacket and a solid top.

I also suggested she buy some jeans in green from Victoria's Secret. They have wonderful colored jeans, and I felt she could get some wear out of them.

Maya's sporty style included some items that were bordering on Trendy, but always with sporty silhouettes.

These are the items Maya added to her daily wardrobe:

1. A pair of emerald jeans (as well as a burgundy pair).
2. Shirts with a more sporty style.
3. I came across a pair of high-top, royal blue sneakers and they reminded me of her. I sent them to her and she loved them. I knew she could wear them as a wardrobe basic.
4. She found a funky surplus-store outfit in burgundy, including a pocket watch. She wore it with a burgundy denim sleeveless blouse. It was a strange combo, but it looked great on her.

5. A ski outfit, in her colors.
6. She already had the daily dresses in her closet. She added a linen dress in burgundy that had buttons down the front, so it also served as a duster.
7. She had plenty of plaid shirts already.
8. Her turtlenecks were old. We added three in burgundy, royal blue, and kelly green.
9. She already had suspenders.
10. She already had a black leather knapsack; we added one in brown.
11. She had one old sports jersey; she added more.
12. She used her cut-off jeans, along with one of the T-shirts I had recommended she use for a cleaning rag, as her new hiking outfit. (Hey, it worked for her.)

Most of my job with Maya was ridding her wardrobe of the items that were too classic and allowing her to make her own decisions about her wardrobe. By the time we finished, she was 100 percent sporty. (By the way, she gave me a psychic reading and it turned out to be pretty accurate. She was right about this book!)

SPORTYS IN THE WORK FORCE

Maya was self-employed. But what if you're not? What if you have an office to go to each day? What if you have sales meetings and presentations?

Sportys are the workhorses of business. They are energetic, moody, and often frazzled.

They're the ones with the messiest office and are frequently the one on the go. They produce near-genius results and no one knows how out of all that clutter.

As a boss, they are wonderful. Since their nature is to be upbeat and supportive, they can spread their cheer.

As an employee, they are intelligent and insightful. While others may tiptoe around an issue, Sportys are frequently able to cut to the heart of the matter.

They are wonderful travel buddies and fun friends, but don't tell them a secret!

Sporty doesn't understand secrets. She's simply not a gossip, and something you told her may find its way into the company newsletter. For no reason other than because she didn't know it was a secret.

Vindictiveness is not in her nature. This is a woman who is a fun coworker.

You must understand that a Sporty is out of her element behind a desk. However, there are many office jobs where she can be active and true to her nature. Since Sportys are competitive, it's no surprise to find them in careers where competition reigns. Always movement for a Sporty!

INTO YOUR CLOSET FOR SPECIAL OCCASIONS

1. White Tie—You may wish to consider renting if this is an infrequent thing for you. If you have no idea where to go, try a tuxedo shop and inquire if they know a place that rents gowns. If you wish to buy, start with a personal shopper at a local department store. On your own, look for pictures of Sporty women in gowns to get ideas.

2. Black Tie—Sporty can wear a man's tuxedo very well.

3. Black Tie Optional—You may need to look at your closet differently to pull out what you already own. One of your longer jackets with a chiffon scarf over a wide-leg pant (or long knit skirt) would work. A pair of your elegant shoes, add a handbag, and you're out the door. This is only one possible combination of many. You're accustomed to seeing your wardrobe in a more casual vein, but if you mix some of your more elegant pieces, the possibilities are endless.

4. Cocktail Reception—Anything goes here, a business suit or a simple dress. Just add

elegant jewelry; real gold or silver earrings, necklace, or bracelet. But don't overload it. Sporty is a very natural style. Too much and it will look overdone. The only addition will be an evening bag, or possibly a pair of heeled shoes, and some fancier earrings.

> **Tip:** If you choose one of the three personal colors in your wardrobe for a special occasion, your accessorizing will be a breeze because you will already own accessories that match your colors.

Are you at a loss as to what to wear to a dance? on a cruise? to a wedding? Then you are definitely a Sporty! But take a gander into your closet first and see what you can come up with.

Pull out a favorite dress that you wear to most occasions. If you have one, it's probably black. Take a look at your collage. Are there any dressy outfits on it?

Now look at the dressy outfit you own. What is the disparity?

Let's do something else here. Where are you going to wear your dressy outfit? Business? If it's a business affair, then you'll want to choose either the color you receive the most compliments on, or the color you feel the most powerful wearing.

Social? Choose the color that you feel is the most like you.

A big presentation? This requires big guns. You may have to use your power color.

Once you have a clear idea of your style and what your needs are, give yourself time to find the outfit. Take time to window shop and browse for what you want. If you don't lose patience, you'll eventually find it.

TOWN OR COUNTRY?

The city Sporty is more sophisticated and polished in her look while maintaining a natural appeal. A country Sporty is more "down to earth" in her persona, still natural, and less polished. Christie Brinkley is an example of a city Sporty, while Julia Roberts is a country Sporty.

Country is easier to buy since her clothes naturally lend themselves to the outdoor lifestyle. But buying versatile fabrics these days makes city life a breeze for Sporty. In fact, of all the style types, she adapts most easily to whatever environment she is in.

SPORTY WARDROBE BASICS

1. A cotton/lycra skirt to wear under sweatshirts or over an animal-print leotard
2. A print leotard you can work out in or wear out
3. A pair of jeans (color is optional)

4. A nice blouse in any fabric or color you choose (I suggest one of your personal colors)
5. A pair of trousers for weekend wear
6. A suit. This may take a while to find. Often, a piece here and a piece there is the best way for you to put together a new suit. A Donna Karan piece with an Esprit or Gap piece can all add up to a fabulous outfit. Suits are not typical attire for you, which is why careful shopping is necessary.
7. A cotton knit outfit, often a long skirt and sweater. Easy to dress up or down.
8. I suggest you always stay on the lookout for special occasion outfits since these are the hardest for you to find. Follow my suggestions for Maya.
9. A Romantic style dress to wear as alternative weekend wear with your tennis shoes

    Note: The focal point of an outfit must be in your style type, but it may not

A SPORTY TRAVELING

Here is a list that my Sporty friend Joie, a flight attendant, compiled of what she packs to travel. On a four-day business trip, all these items should mix and match:

a. One skirt
b. One long vest
c. Two pairs of pants
d. One nice T-shirt
e. One floral dress
f. One dress shirt
g. One blazer
h. One set matching belt, bag, and shoes to go with everything
i. One hat
j. One big T-shirt for sleep
k. One pair tennis shoes
l. One pair tube socks, shorts and T-shirt
m. Four panties, five pairs nylons
n. Two pairs of earrings, two rings, pearls, watch, maybe one scarf
o. A knapsack as a carryall

She packs hot rollers and orders up a blow dryer at the hotel. She also carries two books with her, as she is an avid reader.

As you can see, her business attire has a more relaxed look than those of other style types. Suits don't enter heavily into her wardrobe because she wears a uniform.

(continued)

Let's take a look her list for a seven-day vacation. I asked her to compile a list for a trip to Hawaii. Again, everything for her mixes and matches.

a) one pant
b) one long floral dress
c) one pair jeans
d) one relaxed jacket (a golf-style jacket)
e) two nice T-shirts, one dress shirt
f) one bathing suit, shorts, T-shirt
g) one (each) beach bag and purse

h) one short skirt
i) one pair tennis shoes
j) three pairs tube socks
k) one baseball cap
j) two bras, seven undies
l) one big T-shirt for sleep

She also made a note to me that she'll travel with three or four books for a week's vacation.

To travel to a winter climate, she makes very few substitutions: two sweaters, no skirt, wool socks. She substitutes a coat for her light jacket.

always be the clothes themselves. It can be a watch, a pair of shoes, or earrings.

10. Unobtrusive accessories: a few "sport" watches, one Classic-looking watch to wear with dressier things, and some earrings that work with your personality.

11. Shoes. Make sure you have at least one funky shoe as your basic. Don't play it safe here.

YOUR ACCENT STYLE

As a Sporty woman, you are sparing with your accessories—too many accessories don't really appeal to you.

Romantic

Romantic touches are natural for a Sporty. If this is your accent, then soft feminine touches will make their way into your wardrobe. Long romantic skirts, lace details, and hats will work well on you. A pair of simple dangle earrings could be all you'll need.

Traditional

Traditional elements play a role in many Sporty looks, so this is a natural for a woman who must function in the traditional business world. A Sporty/Traditional may appear almost trendy, at times mixing a sporty skirt with a traditional blazer as an accent. If you wear accessories, they will be understated. Stark and simple is still Sporty.

Classic

Knits will work well for you, and you may find yourself attracted to long lines and classic silhouettes, but steer clear of anything that is too fashion forward, because you may tire of it quickly. The crisp clean look of a Classic clashes with your more relaxed style. Classic sunglasses and watches are accents that won't overpower your ease of style.

Dramatic

While this may seem too much of a contrast, it works as an accent. Anything that you do will have that very important element of "notice me" built in. Your unpretentious style will be infected with a bit of calculation. Dramatic accents here will involve color and a few sexy items.

Trendy

Trendy is the easiest style for you to borrow from because they, too, do the unexpected where accessories are concerned. My friend Joie's watch strap broke and she safety pinned the watch to her dress. Everyone who saw it commented on it. It really did look wonderful, but for her, it was easy and practical—she just didn't have a strap for her watch. Like Trendy, unpretentious; like Sporty, functional.

COLOR WITH YOUR OWN PERSONAL STYLE

Every style type brings her own individual energy to a color. Sporty brings her sense of fair play to whatever color she chooses to wear. Here is the general list of colors as they relate to Sporty. Remember that different shades or hues will vary the meaning, so see the color glossary (Chapter Fourteen) for a fuller meaning.

A Red Outfit

Sporty wears her red in casual attire, but if she puts it on for evening, heads will turn, for red tells others that she loves life, adventure and risk. She may own a red business suit or some fun red accessories, but they are not really her. Red boots and fun red tights can be great. A

Sporty woman will own a red exercise outfit or drive a red sports car. That's where she feels best in red.

An Orange Outfit

Sporty? Orange? Unlike the Dramatic, who doesn't always desire contact, Sporty thrives on it. Sporty's warmth is ignited in orange, where her passion lives. She'll wear orange anywhere, for this is a color that she is *not* afraid to express herself with.

A Yellow Outfit

The element of teamwork is highlighted when Sporty decides to dress in yellow. If she chooses to wear it, she wears it well, for it complements her own physical awareness with an intellectual balance. For Ms. Sporty, there can be an added benefit to wearing yellow: she can be perceived as having intelligence that she's not even aware she has!

A Green Outfit

Whenever having heart and being a good sport counts, you'll find Sporty wearing green. She will show up wearing green when her desire for harmony outweighs her desire to win. A sense of fair play is most important to a Sporty woman.

Whether as a spectator or a participant, you'll see green on a Sporty when she is expressing her feelings of joy. For her, green is more calming and loving than anything else.

A Blue Outfit

A Sporty expresses by doing, not saying, therefore she is out of her element when she must communicate by speaking. She is not as much of a talker as she is a doer, so talking is frequently lost on her. Since Sporty communicates through her physical body, when she wears blue she may be feeling the need to talk things over. When she wears blue she has something to say.

An Indigo Outfit

Ms. Sporty in indigo is exercising a part of herself she is not used to—*her intuition*. A Sporty woman uses her instinct, something that she feels comes from within, rather than an outside source. When a Sporty woman wears indigo, the possibilities are endless. Unlike other style types who may choose indigo naturally, a Sporty woman reaches for it deliberately.

You will find a Sporty woman wearing indigo if:

a) she is making a change in her life and needs to rely upon faith,
b) she needs to let others know that she has matured and come to a decision or new plateau in her life,
c) it looked like navy in the catalog.

A Purple Outfit

A Sporty will select one, perhaps two, shades or hues of purple and shy away from the remainder. The world that a Sporty woman travels in is grounded on this plane; it is incongruent for her to depart for the fantasy life that purple offers her.

However, when Ms. Sporty falls in love, gets married, or has a baby, the elements of purple will enter her wardrobe. For a Sporty can easily get swept up in the emotion of events like these, just as she does with her athletics.

While an impassioned woman (who is very physical), she changes drastically when she gets caught up in her feelings. When her feet leave the ground, *expect* something purple.

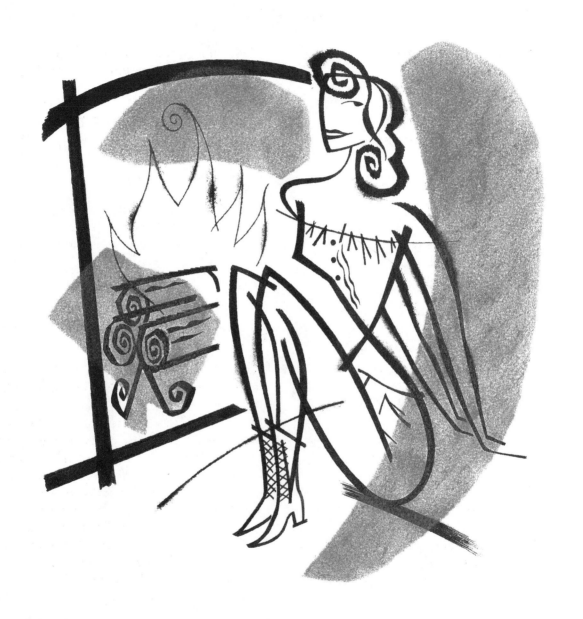

Chapter Five

ROMANTIC

The Romantic woman believes in happily-ever-after and the power of love. In her choice of silhouettes, her clothes reflect a strong femininity.

You may have to travel out of the city to find her, as she is likely to be on a sprawling ranch or large estate (or at the very least, near one). She loves space and often owns land. Although she may be very powerful in her own right, she often willingly plays second to her man. A Romantic marries well, but it may be more than once, since she can easily fall into the fog she calls "love," rather than find the real thing.

It is in later life that a Romantic often finds her prince. She thrives in a relationship and tends to wither without one. The "he" in her life takes top priority, and she almost always dresses for him, hence the Romantic style of elegance, femininity, and sensuality. Romantics do very little struggling, as that is not in their nature. Suffering, however, is in their nature, and they will do plenty of it.

Everything Romantics do is fueled by love. They instinctively pursue what they love and hence hold the secret to success: "If you do what you love, the money will come." To others, a Romantic simply appears to be lucky—as if they have the Midas touch, since almost anything they truly desire comes through for them.

While her demeanor might indicate otherwise, Ms. Romantic works hard, choosing to have a family, career, spouse, and devote herself fully to each of these jobs. In addition to all this, she has charities and other causes to which she feels a special kinship.

Because it is passion that impels her forward, at times she could seem too controlling or abrasive to others. But most of those around her know how deeply she loves them and that is all consuming to her. Having love in her life is of primary importance to her, and she never seems to be without it. Romantics can sometimes float from one relationship to the next, not quite realizing how they did it. It's not that they can't live without love, it's just that it finds them, because the amount of love and passion they exude draws others to them.

The designs that best reflect a Romantic woman have a floral, lace, and frilly flowing style that says "romance."

RECOGNIZING A ROMANTIC

Marilyn Monroe. Yes. No, she's not a Dramatic. Her whole life wasn't about making an entrance, although she certainly stirred things up when she walked into a room. But a Dramatic would never appear less than perfect in public and Marilyn often did, especially when she was emotionally distraught. Marilyn was a true Romantic, searching for love and successful naturally.

Marilyn's famous pose over the subway grating as she pushed down her billowing skirt showed her sensuality. That was pure Romantic.

Jennifer Beals, a Romantic, was well matched to the Romantic Alex in *Flashdance*. In the movie, she talks about feeling the music, is driven by her feelings, and puts her passions above all else.

Remember: a Romantic woman is sensual and emotional, on the opposite side of the wheel from Dramatic; she is the counterbalance to Dramatic's strong, bold, sexy message.

What are the elements that make an outfit romantic?

The warmth and gentleness of a Romantic woman touch everyone who comes in contact with her. While to some she may not appear passionate or driven, when it comes to love, nothing can stop her. When a romantic wears a sweater, it could be a crocheted one (with the look of feminine lace). A bold cuff bracelet could appear to be from another style type, but it is a definite romantic accessory. Not everything off the shoulder is romantic, but a relaxed and sensual look is Romantic. A peasant or poet's blouse can be part of your natural grace. Old-fashioned granny boots are very romantic.

> **Tip:** Remember, we all easily tire of things that are not our style type. So make sure the key items you buy are in your style type.

A Romantic can wear jewelry that would appear gaudy on others, but on her it's sexy and spectacular. At times, a Romantic can appear almost bohemian; there is a definite element of it to anything she wears. Remember, she throws everything to the wind for love, and she will risk anything for it.

The soft line is always the key for a Romantic woman. Look for soft flowing fabrics to indicate a romantic silhouette.

A ROMANTIC STORY

Once upon a time, there lived a young woman who was quite miserable. Her life was nothing like she wanted it to be, and she felt that a change of clothing would help her. Unfortunately, her problem went much deeper than mere clothing. It was life-style, too. When she discovered that it was "romance" that was missing from her life, she found herself and lived happily ever after.

It's very common for a Romantic to live her life in the wrong style type. When Gwen came to me, it was via a mutual friend who was a career counselor. Gwen was a real estate lawyer, and the firm she worked for was very traditional. She wore a floral suit that did not mesh with the office atmosphere, and her office looked like a rain forest. Plants hung everywhere, and in the middle of the shrubbery was a massive mahogany desk that resembled something from the nineteenth century. It occurred to me that she must be excellent at her job or the firm never would have kept such a mismatch around.

Gwen plopped behind her desk and sighed. She was miserable. At the top of her firm, in line for partnership, and she couldn't stand it. In her own words, she "felt out of place." As with Romantics, there is a story behind her misery.

Gwen had a professor in college whom she adored. They had an affair. He went to a law school to teach, and she applied there so they could remain together. They did. She married him and they had a child.

By the time they divorced, she had her law degree and was already practicing. Gwen had missed the opportunity to choose her career; love had chosen it for her.

Her secret desire was to move to another country and live on a farm. As she told me about her dream of opening a knitting salon, her eyes sparkled. Only her intercom buzz forced her back to reality.

While she was on the phone, I took a minute to size up the situation. She was definitely a Romantic. Her driving force was love, and she could not possibly find any happiness unless she followed her heart.

The quiz also revealed that she was a Romantic. I had an instinct about what that meant, but I couldn't say anything about it yet (since I suspected it involved a job and location change). As I watch my clients go through the quiz, collage, and statement, they often get to discover for themselves what may be obvious to their friends and the rest of the world.

CLOSET OR COLLAGE?

Gwen's collage helped her really see what mattered to her. After she discovered that she was a Romantic, her world began to blossom.

On her collage were soft, flowing skirts, crocheted knit tops, rings, and hair that was soft and natural.

The pictures she clipped for the background were all from grassy knolls, country lanes or quaint shops and resembled a New England town. I made a mental note of this before we moved on.

When we discussed her collage, she herself was surprised by the outcome. Gwen was beginning to comprehend why she had never felt fulfilled.

In her own words, she "went from my mother's house to my husband's." She always followed love, never really following her own mind.

As we set to work on her wardrobe, she began to consider where she'd like to live. I pointed out my earlier observation: the New England setting of her collage.

This surprised her. She'd loved Boston when she'd once visited there. It began to feel right to her.

I suggested she write her statement before making any decisions. Her written statement brought more clarity to her. She had dreamed of living on a farm in the south of France, but with a child still in school, Boston held much more for her.

But first, we decided a closet clearing was in order.

COLORS IN HER CLOSET

Gwen had spent a fortune several years before hiring a woman to coordinate her wardrobe. By the looks of her closet, the woman she had hired was a Traditional. The two style types are close enough so that a Romantic woman like Gwen wouldn't have known that she was being led down the wrong path. Almost half of the silhouettes in her closet were incorrect. Her former fashion consultant did get her seasonal colors right. She was an "autumn", and in cleaning out her closet, we found her three personal colors.

1. Pumpkin was the color she felt best wearing (how she sees herself),
2. Olive was the color she received the most compliments in (how the world sees her), and
3. Dark cocoa was her power color.

The colors were all there in her closet.

Before you read my conclusions, try this: look up each of Gwen's colors in the color glossary (Chapter Fourteen) and consider the extra information you know about Gwen. The colors at the end of this chapter will give you a general idea of how your style can vary the meaning of a color slightly. Confer with the glossary for specific colors, but this general overview is tailored for your style.

Now, let's go back to Gwen, beginning with the color she feels best wearing— pumpkin. This tells me she is sincere and fair. She is also interested in others' well-being; this is *not* a selfish woman.

Olive is the color she receives the most compliments on. The world sees this woman as dependable and very capable.

And finally, dark cocoa brown tells me that she derives her energy from being true to herself on a very deep level.

Why is color important here? What does this tell me? Consider the additional information we now have about Gwen. I know she's going to follow through on the work we do together, because she carefully considers whatever she undertakes.

I also know that personal contact is important to her. This is a clue to the way I can approach creating her shopping list with her.

THE SHOPPING LIST

First, we had to go through everything and figure out what was going to stay in her closet from her Traditional personal shopper.

She owned three new, very traditional blazers. These would have to be replaced, but we opted to use them over floral dresses and challis skirts for the time being. They were simply too traditional to wear on their own.

We also found a few very traditional slacks, and they had matching blouses. Colors right; style wrong. We opted to find a few Romantic blouses to wear with the slacks, and the blouses (which she didn't really like) she gave to a local charity.

My first plan of attack was to list the items that were going to first need to be replaced. She needed to diversify what she already had in her closet. Since I knew her plan was to move to New England within a year, we searched for romantic pieces that would work in her new environment.

1. She needed at least one romantic blazer. I suggested a long blazer with a shawl collar in olive.
2. A brown jacket, long or short
3. A long dress that flows
4. A short soft skirt (in a pattern to go with her traditional blazers as well as her new Romantic acquisitions)
5. A lace top, again to soften the traditional blazer
6. Bodysuits (in her 3 colors) plus mustard and rust
7. Two sweaters, one crocheted in oyster (to wear over her bodysuit with either leggings or a skirt)
8. A KMO (Knock me over) bulky cable knit sweater for her frequent ski trips
9. Ballet shoes in olive for weekend wear
10. Woven sandals for summer
11. A soft satchel bag for a purse

As the traditional pieces wore out or she no longer wore them, she was instructed to not replace them, but to find their romantic sisters instead. Gwen felt fabulously comfortable with the idea of dressing in her style type.

THE RESULTS

1. Gwen's local department store had the perfect olive blazer. It was a 1940s silhouette in lightweight gabardine.

2. The brown jacket she spotted at a local boutique. It was a cotton interlock sweater with puffed sleeves that looked like a short bolero jacket. She called me and asked me if I thought the style was right and could be substituted. Perfect! It would work with everything she owned and was great for those more relaxed days at the office or for dressy casual wear.

3. She splurged and bought a few long dresses. One was a sleeveless gabardine in greige (gray-beige) that was exquisite. She also found a gold cuff bracelet.

She also bought a floral in pumpkin, moss green, and brown. This was a silk, and while it had no hanger appeal, on her, with her pounded-gold cuff bracelet and matching earrings, it looked exquisite.

This could also be doubled as her "day-wedding guest" dress. I suggested she buy a sexy strappy sandal for summer events. She agreed and found one in brown.

4. She bought a silk skirt (above the knee) in a salmon/jade floral. It worked beautifully with her new brown knit jacket/sweater.

5. A lace bodysuit in camel that matched one of her traditional blazers, and worked with her new floral skirt.

6. She found all 5 of the colors on her list in bodysuits. She also splurged on a turquoise one for her denim skirt.

7. She found the long crocheted sweater in oyster at her local department store. The cable knit sweater she found in a thrift store. She bought it in terra cotta.

8. Cuff bracelets in both a pounded gold and a flat gold that had matching earrings available. When we got to the store, she confessed that she didn't like silver, so we opted for the gold only.

9. There were olive tennis shoes, and they would work with quite a bit in her closet. There was also a 1½-inch-heel pump in brown and it looked so good on her, she bought it.

10. Dark brown woven sandals—she'd get years of wear out of these.

11. A soft mini duffel bag. This soft shape defies the more structured shapes that Traditional would wear.

As a result of our working together, Gwen made her own additions to her daily wardrobe:

1. A brown stirrup (heavyweight for fall) pant. She could use her new brown sweater with a gold cuff bracelet and matching jewelry.
2. A poet's blouse
3. Low-heeled jodhpur boots in dark brown
4. A new belt, brown with a gold buckle
5. A long cotton sweater in chartreuse. This would also go over her brown leggings.

Much of the job with Gwen, as it is with many Romantics, was to rid her wardrobe of past "love interests."

The men in a Romantic woman's life are a great influence. I have a friend who was distraught when she and her rock musician boyfriend broke up. Not because the relationship was over, but because she'd bought so many outfits to please him.

Ms. Romantic will dress to match her man more than another style type will. Unfortunately, when the affair is over, she's left with a wardrobe that doesn't match.

Incidentally, Gwen and her daughter did move to Boston, and Gwen opened a small law practice. I understand she's doing quite well.

they do. They don't subscribe to the all-black school because to them all black is devoid of feeling, not at all Ms. Romantic's thing.

ROMANTICS IN THE WORK FORCE

A Romantic at work is a hard worker who aims to please. Soft, feminine, and emotionally driven wouldn't necessarily be the description of a successful executive. But don't be fooled by Romantic's femininity! She's a tiger, able and unafraid of working among the most powerful of men.

Her strong vulnerability opens many doors for her, for she learned long ago that she must be herself. Above all else, she loves men. And she isn't afraid to be a woman.

You can easily find a Romantic in an office, but more than likely she is involved in the arts in some way. She can be a whiz at administrative jobs and is at ease being the power behind the throne.

Competition is not Ms. Romantic's element, harmony is, so look for her to be involved in anything that is emotionally comforting.

Her clothes, like her career, must be comfortable and make her feel good.

Romantics aren't afraid to wear color, and

INTO YOUR CLOSET FOR SPECIAL OCCASIONS

For a Romantic, colors need to define her, not a fabricated image. Bold is good for a Dramatic, for it matches her personality. A Romantic needs to blend with her clothes, and they should appear as a part of her sensuality.

For her, the era doesn't really matter. Nineteen fifties Marilyn Monroe or present day.

1. White Tie—

This is hard to just pull out of your closet because it is so formal, and unless you go to quite a few white-tie events, you might not have anything suitable. This is definitely a return to a more Romantic era. A sexy, tight-fitting floor-length gown would be you, as would a more traditional ball gown cut slightly lower than a Traditional would feel comfortable wearing. Do pick one of your three personal colors to make a statement, or a color that you feel magnificent in. The orange family is the most powerful for you.

2. Black Tie—

This type of event is ultrafeminine for you. An elegantly draped silk dress would work here. Romantics can border on Dramatic at times with formal wear. Here are a few tips to avoid the obvious pitfalls:

a) Make sure the outfit is sensual, not sexy (it's okay to be both, just focus on sensual).
b) Fabric can move or cling. Remember Marilyn Monroe in her skin-tight dresses? Her sexiness was not bold and forceful like a Dramatic, but innocent unassuming like a Romantic.
c) Don't wear white-tie formal, keep yourself in the present day.

3. Black Tie Optional—

I recently saw a Romantic woman wearing some "Santa Fe" accessories, a peasant blouse, and a sheer skirt with a catsuit underneath. Now to some, this look may be dated, but she looked fabulous. It was her style!

A ROMANTIC TRAVELING

My best friend Linda is a producer, and she would kill me if I didn't use her packing list. Whenever I pick her up at the airport, it requires an extra cart. Romantics in general don't understand the concept of packing light.

Here is her list for a Four-Day business trip:

a) A soft, classically styled suit with a subtle flower pattern. (This is for major "corporate"-type meetings.)
b) A circle skirt, floral pattern, voile, two layers. Two different tops to match.
c) One pair brown plaid pants (wide leg now; narrow if wide is out)
d) One black turtleneck if it's winter; silk campshirt if summer.
e) Two pairs of black panty hose, for after hours
f) One pair sage palazzo pants
g) Yellow tank top with lace neckline
h) One flowered "baby doll" dress, very short
i) One pair of low-heeled black pumps (for most business outfits)
j) One pair of sage mules
k) One pair of sneakers
l) One gym outfit (unitard shorts)
m) T-shirt
n) hair dryer and travel-size toiletries

P.S: Her Traditional mother packs everything in plastic bags; not just shoes—*everything!*

(*continued*)

Here is Linda's list for a seven-day trip to the Islands

a) One white bikini
b) One-piece bathing suit (need to purchase)
c) Large batik cloth for wrapping (as a skirt/sarong/coverup)
d) Black top with lace trim
e) A button-front dress in a muted yellow floral pattern
f) Sage flowered palazzo pants
g) Yellow tank T-shirt w/lace neckline
h) Two to three workout outfits
i) One pair linen gray shorts
j) Black tank top
k) Pink linen jacket
l) Sage green mules
m) White crocheted flats
n) Black lace-up sandals
o) Sneakers
p) Two short sundresses
q) Two sets matching bra/panties (sexy!)
r) One short negligee
s) Sunblock
t) Walkman with "beach" tapes
u) Two to three books for beach reading
v) Fanny pack for beach trips and exercise outings
w) Hair dryer
x) My man goes with me. Second choice, my best friend.

ROMANTIC WARDROBE BASICS

Much of your work will be in reclaiming your style. There are a few things to be on the look-out for:

1. Another flowing romantic dress, in a color right for you
2. A sheer blouse, to go over a bodysuit or camisole
3. A new hat. Something with ribbons or flowers. Hair ornaments are also important for you. Be careful to stay romantic and not get too traditional. (There is a raw, unpolished element to a Romantic. Remember: go bohemian before polished!)
4. Dangle earrings. Also, don't forget bracelets.
5. Shoes. A new pair of T-straps or new espadrilles, depending upon your focus, "work" or casual. Ballet shoes are always an option for you.

6. A fantabulous bag is also on the list. Something lace or cloth.
7. A pair of lace gloves for tea or special occasions
8. A soft pastel dress to wear to a bridal shower, a christening, or a *bris*. You, like the Traditional woman, get invited to plenty of gatherings.
9. A new suit, bought at the right time of year—find the appropriate color and fabric weight for your needs. You'll need something with a peplum top or embroidery. Remember feminine *details*.
10. Casual weekend wear is usually lacking. This is mostly because your whole life is lived with an air of romance about it (we all tend to overlook the obvious). A pair of men's chinos to wear with a great sun hat and sneakers is a romantic weekend look.
11. A poet's blouse to wear with jeans

The most important thing is how you feel in the clothes you wear. I know, all of us like our clothes to feel right, but most women will purchase something if it looks great. You won't. You have to *feel* great in the outfit, and that is more important than a look; we'll work on both.

YOUR ACCENT STYLE

Many other style types have come and taken from you over the years. Let's see what *you* can take from *them*.

Sporty

A Romantic can freely use Sporty elements, for she would never lose her feminine looks. No matter how casual she may be dressed, Romantic will always maintain her soft side. The elements of Sporty that she loves are already ingrained in her personality.

If Sporty is your accent, the things you are best suited for are outdoor sports like horseback riding. You are not afraid of being feminine no matter what, and others respect your determination to excel at whatever you undertake.

This is a very brave accent.

Romantic

Romantics need to simply wear their own accent pieces. Dangle earrings, cuff bracelets, jewelry, and even rings. Remember that even in business settings, wearing purely your own style type is very powerful.

Traditional

This is the style that falls right after Romantic and therefore adds an upscale element to Romantic. The blending of these two can, at times, give the appearance of a Trendy, because the look seems so unique.

Traditional touches on a Romantic do add a conservative air to a free spirit, and you may want to keep an eye on the details you choose. Don't overdo this.

Classic

Jane Seymour is a perfect Romantic/Classic. With her polish and sense of style, she can carry off some beautiful classic pieces. But, it is her ability to make us identify with romance and a more gentle time that makes her a pure Romantic. In the roles that have made her famous, she created characters who were tortured by love, and yet were the object of great love.

Jane Seymour's purity of style and the sense that she would risk the things most precious to her for love, have made her a successful miniseries star.

Accent carefully, for a Classic is in some ways too modern for you and may dilute some of the charm of your style.

Dramatic

Dramatic accents on a Romantic woman is a volatile combination. Vivian Leigh was a Romantic whose accent was on the Dramatic. She was a woman who was driven by love and made all her choices based on her feelings. Her dramatic beauty was heightened when she wore her pure romantic clothing. Look at her most memorable role: Scarlett O'Hara. A woman driven by love, but needing to be the center of attention. If this is your accent, you know how to draw attention to yourself and keep it. Whatever you wear, it will be soft, feminine, and brazen. With a dramatic accent, you use bold colors or dramatic accessories to be a show stopper.

Trendy

Trendy is actually quite a common accent for Ms. Romantic. She will blend funky pieces with those of a more romantic time. She is the woman who isn't afraid to break rules that are considered unbreakable.

A Romantic can mix any style in with hers. The only drawback here is that if she dilutes herself too much, she will bury her romantic style.

Don't let a trendy accent make you such a renegade that you forget your core. Make sure that the focal point of your outfit is always romantic.

COLOR WITH YOUR OWN PERSONAL STYLE

Romantic brings the element of love to whatever color she chooses to wear.

A Red Outfit

Red itself carries a pure sexual and passionate energy which overpowers the softness of a Romantic. Muted versions of red are best since they won't contradict the soft message she wants to send out. A red suit is not congruent with her style. Besides, a Romantic

woman wears her red underneath it all, in lingerie!

An Orange Outfit

A Romantic gently inspires others with her consistency, and orange is well placed with her. (When she is feeling the need to nestle in her home, you may find some of the shades and hues of orange around the house.)

Her warmth is typically physical, therefore this is where Ms. Romantic's sexual energy is sparked. Her thoughts have turned toward her partner when she selects something in the orange family to wear.

She'll wear orange out on a date, to a wedding, or to a romantic dinner. She'll wear something in the orange family anytime she's *feeling* romantic.

A Yellow Outfit

Always subtle, always gentle. That is how Ms. Romantic wears her yellow. Regardless of shade or hue, she never seeks to show off her intelligence. For this simply is not important to her. Her thinking is original and is always done in a softspoken way. At times, her intelligence often surprises those around her.

She'll show up in a yellow outfit at her next meeting, throwing everyone so off guard with her choice of color that she can't help but make a statement!

A Green Outfit

Like the tiny leaves on a baby tree, Ms. Romantic sweeps in with an air of hope and renewal. She reaches for green when she is feeling rejuvenated and connected to her current love.

This may be a new relationship, project, or cause. Ms. Romantic lives in a world where peace and harmony are paramount to her success; since peace and harmony are what green is all about, rarely will she have a lack of green in her wardrobe.

Expect to see her wearing green to be a spectator at the races, for this is her color of enjoyment and freedom.

A Blue Outfit

A Romantic woman is loyal no matter what. Her faith is unwavering and often the cornerstone of her life.

She communicates this to others whenever she slips into something blue. More than any other style type, a Romantic's mood is dictated by the hue or shade she chooses. She is moody, and her moods can also be easily influenced by the blue that others around her choose to wear.

An Indigo Outfit

Interestingly, indigo and the Romantic are mismatched energies. A Romantic derives energy from being grounded to the earth, while indigo pulls it from above.

A Romantic needs to feel grounded, and pure indigo (unless it is mixed with brown) can make her feel off balance and out of sorts.

Rarely will a Romantic choose a solid indigo—for her power source comes from the earth, to which *she* feels spiritually connected. Her intuition is strongly related to earthly matters.

A Purple Outfit

The lofty and distinguished quality of purple is not lost with Ms. Romantic. When she selects purple, her mood is in synch with the shade she chooses. Like nibbling on her favorite chocolate bar, she loves to indulge in purple, which is all about enjoyment of beauty.

Ms. Romantic wears purple when she wishes to rise above a possibly volatile situation, yet remain centered and calm within. She may wear purple to a divorce proceeding.

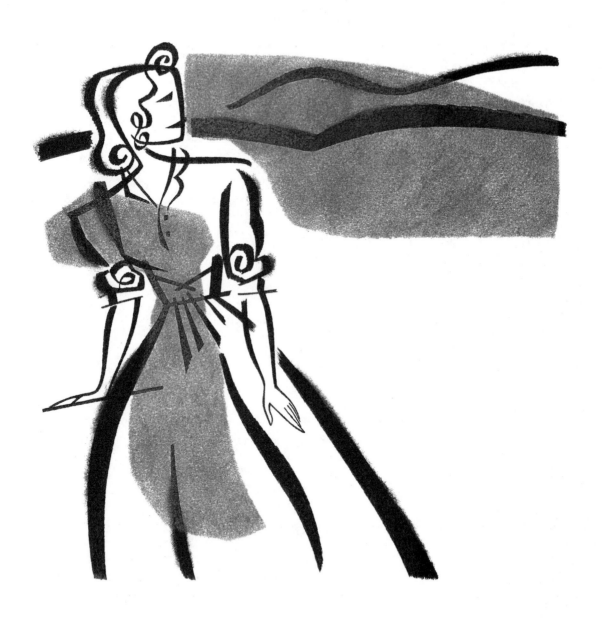

Chapter Six

TRADITIONAL

Famous Traditionals

Ellen Barkin, Barbara Bush, Hillary Rodham Clinton, Princess Diana, Mia Farrow, Florence Henderson, Helen Hunt, Coretta Scott King, Angela Lansbury, Mary Tyler Moore, Jane Pauley, Eleanor Roosevelt, Sissy Spacek, Meryl Streep, Patricia Wettig

Traditional Focus:

Tradition

Traditional Quote:

"Courtesy costs nothing, yet it buys things that are priceless."

The Traditional woman is deeply sensitive and kind. She is by nature a good listener and a caring friend. She'll easily draw you into a conversation, then about an hour later you'll realize that she's said nothing about herself.

Giving to a fault, a Traditional goes above and beyond for others. She remembers the birthdays that her Classic sister forgets, and often maintains one solid marriage throughout her life.

There isn't much this woman won't do for those she loves. She is an ideal partner in work or life and is adored by friends and loved ones. She's the one who marks her calendar with birthdays. Don't be surprised to find her on committees to help decorate for parties or pouring punch at the PTA.

This woman finds the elderly precious and chooses to care for them when others would give up on them. Traditional women have the patience of saints.

America is on the whole a traditional country, and Traditional is without a doubt the most-often-found style type in the United

States. The "preppie" look in the early 1980s can attest to that! Preppie is another aspect of a Traditional.

A Traditional is a one-man woman, a fabulous companion, and a wonderful inspiration. Most men will tell you that *their* mother is a Traditional.

She has a deep hankering for a family and the responsibilities that go with it. She will do whatever has to be done to be of service to others. Always the first to ask to help, she is a friend to be counted on. This is the woman who is loyal, trustworthy, and gets the job done without complaining.

She rarely buys any "fake" or costume jewelry. She truly appreciates genuine pearls and wears them well. Although she wears nice clothes, they are rarely high fashion—she prefers to splurge on her loved ones.

She is the first to buy a dependable-name product over a bargain brand, however, as this is a woman who appreciates fine workmanship, buying the best quality and knowing that it'll last.

Pendleton is one example of the many labels that reflect the Traditional woman.

RECOGNIZING A TRADITIONAL

Actress Meryl Streep is a Traditional. While one of her early movies, *Kramer vs. Kramer*, didn't show her in the most positive light, it did show a Traditional woman's torture over leaving her child. This is also a marvelous example of matching a Traditional woman to a traditional role.

Traditional Sissy Spacek in her Oscar-winning role as country singer Loretta Lynn in the movie *Coal Miner's Daughter* was perfectly matched to the character she portrayed. Mia Farrow in the classic film *Rosemary's Baby* was a Traditional also perfectly matched to the role she played.

In general we tend to go to the movies for plot, and television to see characters we care about each week, so it's no surprise to find that Traditional women are all over the tube.

A Traditional's style is basic American clothing, and Florence Henderson as the mom on "The Brady Bunch," portrayed the typical Traditional mother. Who will ever forget Mrs. Brady? Her whole style was traditional, her hair, the clothes, but most of all the caring and concern she felt for her children and husband. She was the mother of an entire generation of kids.

Another generation lived vicariously each week through Mary Richards' life as a single working woman on "The Mary Tyler Moore Show." Who can deny that this endearing Traditional woman didn't matter to all of us?

Patricia Wettig in "thirtysomething" was

a perfect Traditional. (No, sorry, the part of Hope played by Mel Harris was a Classic. Why? Her anxiety was over her career. Different focus.)

Helen Hunt is among the newest generation of Traditional women. Her outspoken style is refreshing, and her deep concern and caring for others never leave her in any role she plays.

Traditional women do tend to be the most popular on television, because the American public can easily relate to them. Yes, she is the easiest to spot, the best friend to have, and the easiest to buy clothing for.

In the next section, we'll take a look at a few silhouettes that are typically Traditional.

What are the elements that make an outfit traditional?

The understated simplicity of a garment signifies Traditional. Plain and simple is what works best for her, illustrating her high standards. For a Traditional, basics are best and no one wears them better than she does. While other style types will have a focal point to their outfits, Traditional generally won't because each piece is a basic, and all her pieces add up to the same simple statement. This actually makes dressing easier for her. While other style types build out from basics, Traditional's clean wholesome image is built on it. Any accessories she chooses are most likely pearls or a delicate brushed gold.

Traditional and Sporty can appear to run very close in terms of silhouettes, and while a relaxed pant can easily be worn by a Sporty, the jackets Traditionals like are often too tailored for Ms. Sporty.

Every few seasons, Trendys and Classics grab onto the simplicity of a Traditional and with a few spare accessories they turn Traditional into a new trend. While a basic long skirt (or longer shorts) with a T-shirt and loafers may go in and out, for Traditional they are always in, and most of the time found in her closet. Plaids and florals are both traditional.

Whenever the fashions turn to American style, the spotlight is on traditional looks first. The simple becomes highlighted and the pieces in a traditional wardrobe become chic, much to the chagrin of this woman, who doesn't understand what all the fuss is about. She has, after all, been wearing quality fabrics and understated styles for years. Dresses are very important to Traditionals and many dress styles are traditional. Traditionals tend to reach for separates quite a bit. A matching skirt and blouse ensemble that can go from day to dinner is a staple for most Traditionals. There is a timeless charm to a Traditional woman.

A TRADITIONAL STORY

When I met Rose, she was not only reentering the work force, she was reentering life. Her husband of thirty years had recently passed away, and her life had changed almost overnight. With her daughters' help, she decided to rebuild her wardrobe, but there were two problems.

The first was her Classic daughter, Annette. Rose didn't feel comfortable with Annette's choices for her. In her zeal to redo Mom, Annette chose some fashion-forward classic styles that were simply not Rose.

Her second problem was her Dramatic daughter, Michelle, who added dramatic hats and gloves that actually "wore" Rose. Dramatic styles simply outshine a Traditional and don't flatter her at all.

By the time she reached me, Rose was completely demoralized. (As will happen if you're trying on clothes that aren't in your style type. You will begin to feel as though nothing will work on you.) It's even worse if others around you try on the same outfit and look great. Try to keep in mind that if someone else looks sensational in an outfit and you don't, it's probably not your style.

Rose hadn't focused on her wardrobe in years—and had no idea where to start. To keep

her sanity and her relationship with her daughters intact, she hired me.

I didn't need to see her quiz results to know she was a Traditional in every sense of the word.

Regardless, the quiz was taken, and the results were as I suspected. She was a pure Traditional and would have to stay away from other style-type accents.

A pure style type is really quite striking. She is the woman whose manner takes all the positive qualities of her style type and magnifies them. In the case of a Traditional, it's hard to avoid seeing how kind, loving, and unselfish she truly is.

On a pure style type (Traditional is most commonly a pure type), accenting with another style will not only look out of place, it will feel awkward as well.

Being a pure Traditional is very easy to dress for. Quite a few catalogs cater to the Traditional woman, and her simple styling is fun to shop for.

CLOSET OR COLLAGE?

Rose had a set way she wanted to work with me. Her idea was to go through the whole process and then wait to buy. Rose wanted to lose ten pounds before buying new clothes. When I found out that she had been a size fourteen for almost twenty years, I told her that I couldn't work that way. My feeling was that we should do everything. She finally agreed with the stipulation that she could stop at any time (that is a client's right). She showed up first with her collage. I found this interesting since I'd recommend that she first do a statement, but her collage proved very revealing.

Rose had a fuller figure and all the pictures in her collage were of women who were tiny! I mean thinner than is healthy. The current trend in the modeling industry is to use models who are so thin they look nothing like real women. Rose had picked the correct fashions, but the pictures didn't resemble her in any way.

Then, I did something that I'd never done before. I suggested she get some magazines and catalogs of larger-sized women and make another collage out of that. Her images of what she should look like were simply disproportionate to who she was. First of all, Rose was a big-boned woman, and anything below a size ten wouldn't be becoming on her.

Redoing her collage opened a floodgate for her. This collage had more images of healthy, sexy, fuller women who were active and attractive. This was more current and appropriate for Rose.

This time I was struck by how she personally didn't wear much color, but her collage was filled with soft summer tones. There was no doubt in my mind that she was drawn to these colors because they looked best on her.

The pictures in her second collage reflected her desire to reenter the job market. She'd left a job as an administrator at a law firm when she had her second child and hadn't seen a paycheck with her name on it for many years. This was something she now wanted very badly.

The second collage also gave her permission to be the size she was.

Her statement provided clues that would be important later. In it she wrote how she wanted to "brighten" up her life. She didn't want to be somber any longer. While she missed her husband, she didn't want to remain in the dark and mourn him forever. This woman was ready to remake herself, which is uncharacteristic of a Traditional, who is not usually comfortable with changes. I made a mental note of this discrepancy.

Then I got the phone call. She felt that the whole process had worked beautifully for her, but she'd decided that she wanted to run with her newfound knowledge.

I knew that the work was only halfway there, but there isn't much you can do to convince a client (who is paying you) to continue on. So I told her to stay in touch and let me know how she was doing.

Unfortunately, in her rush to save herself a few steps, she fell into a common problem that many Traditional women tend to make;

they buy the same silhouettes and miss out on the versatility available to them in purchasing things they normally wouldn't consider. Rose made a list and off she went to shop.

To illustrate the problem, let's begin with her list.

1. A pantsuit for daywear
2. Two new suits to mix with blouses she already owns
3. Three blouses to wear with her new suits
4. One new dress (for work and social functions)
5. One casual pant

Rose had neglected to clean out her closet, so when she came home with her new acquisitions, she jammed them into an already full wardrobe. She said she stared at her bulging wardrobe for almost an hour before she called me with an SOS.

She had decided that new suits were her answer. She wound up with two suits that she liked, but this was the way she had shopped for years. There was no delineation between her looks. Suits had always been worn for volunteer things, church occasions, and evenings out with her husband. And, quite frankly, her purchases were dated. While the colors were fine, she had two suits that were nothing special.

Luckily, I received the call before she snipped the tags.

I glanced at her list on my way to her closet. Her entire wardrobe was filled with dark somber clothes and her new purchases were black, navy, and taupe. In addition, many of the things were very dramatic in their styling. As I looked her closet, my memory of the inconsistencies in her collage and statement came back to me. She had used the word *somber* to describe her husband. I guessed that he was a Dramatic, and when she showed me his picture, I was correct. Since he loved to see her in his favorite colors, he was probably a winter.

That wasn't completely off, since they shared a few colors, but over the years she had got lost in his style and found herself unable to distinguish what she was buying for herself and what was for him. On top of all this, she liked his style, as many women do, because the Dramatic man can be very dashing!

But it wasn't Rose.

My job with her was beginning to get more difficult! It's easy when a woman buys her own clothes, then I know what colors she is drawn to, but in her case what stood before me was a massive closet filled with her husband's favorite colors.

My eyes fell on her collage. There before me was a whole bunch of colors that Rose liked. Pay dirt! Almost all of them fell onto the "summer" wheel.

We proceeded slowly and hung, sorted, and stored her clothing.

COLORS IN HER CLOSET

In Rose's case, it took slightly longer than usual, but we found her three personal colors. They were:

1. Rose, the color, was what she felt best wearing (how she sees herself),
2. Baby blue was the color she received the most compliments on (how the world sees her), and
3. Rich cranberry was the color she felt powerful wearing.

The truth regarding what was going on with Rose was hidden in the colors that emerged as her personal colors. Before you read on, go take a look at the book's glossary (Chapter Fourteen) and see what you can discern about Rose yourself. According to her colors, Rose is a detail-oriented person but doesn't get much opportunity to display her organizational skills. She is excellent at organizing her family; this is apparent in her choice of rose for the color she feels best wearing.

The baby blue tells me that others perceive her as the perfect problem solver. She easily deals with situations creatively and equitably. Since baby blue does not project authority, others are not threatened by it. While she has very capable analytic skills, she knows how to blend in to not intimidate others who are less capable than she.

And finally, cranberry turns out to be a very revealing choice for her power color! She is able to trust her instincts and be very forward about her ambitions. (This is probably why she was able to stay married to a Dramatic man for so many years. This was a woman who knows how to speak her mind if she needs to.)

After discovering her personal colors, which confirmed my initial instinct about Rose, I had a good idea of how to approach a wardrobe.

Rose already owned a few suits, and she asked me to help her work with what was already there. I agreed. My goal was to widen her options with as minimal a cost as possible, and in so doing, fully utilize what was already hanging in her closet.

One of the easiest ways to cut costs when building a wardrobe is to work with your personal colors.

Luckily, Rose already owned quite a few pieces in her personal colors, and we set to work on her list.

THE SHOPPING LIST

Rose felt comfortable with the idea of a suit, but it wasn't necessarily right for her. I also had to consider that she had once been a size eight, but for the better part of the last twenty years she had been a size fourteen. Not large by any stretch of the imagination, in fact, it is an average size.

There were a few other benefits to Rose's size. The first thing was that if she shopped in the women's section of her local department stores, she was bound to find lots of values. Many women who are size fourteen shop in the missy sizes. This is purely ego, and they wind up spending more money. The bonus to being a fourteen is that many nice fashions can be found on the mark-down racks in women's since that is the size that is the border between women's and missy.

Lucky fourteens!

With all this in mind, I knew it wouldn't be too hard to find her a few items to get her wardrobe started.

There was much that we weeded out of her wardrobe. Anything that did not currently fit her and had not fit her for over a year was history! Almost half of her bulging closet had been a size eight or ten. A few things still had tags on! Parting with her "somedays" was painful for her.

We wound up with a new shopping list for Rose.

1. An elegant suit. We'd wait for something traditional in any of her personal colors. We were going to make this a building block for an interview ensemble.

2. A pantsuit in her rich cranberry color
3. Going all the way, a blouse in cocoa or brown, to match her cranberry suit
4. Two summer dresses in her pastel colors
5. Two cool-climate dresses, one in her pastels, one in plum or emerald (from the summer color wheel)
6. A summer suit that she could wear to a wedding or church, then use for work later on
7. Two blazers, one in a pastel print and one in a deep tone, either a solid neutral or a pattern to go with her vast collection of darker pieces. This darker toned blazer was to bring together her colors and utilize the many items she already owned.
8. Three pairs of slacks that fit her, in any of the neutrals that are on her palette: navy, gray, off-white, taupe, cocoa, and tan. Yes, she had owned pants, but they were too small for her. This accounted for her belief that pants never looked good on her. She'd never actually owned any pants that fit her.
9. A few basic turtlenecks that were on sale (for the following fall). She was to pick a few bright colors from the summer color wheel.
10. A few silk or polyester shells to mix and match with her new suits.

She thought she already had suits, but by the time we'd cleared out her closet she only had one left that fit her, in navy. We had another goal: to do all this slowly.

Rose did have many pieces that were easy to make work. Once she saw her clothes in color order, she herself began to imagine new combinations. Her grays and browns now blended beautifully with the new pastels.

THE RESULTS

Something happened to Rose after we made up her list and cleared out her closet. Her needs were clear to her, and she didn't have any problems finding things that worked for her. I had become fond of Rose and accompanied her on a few of her expeditions.

Here is what she actually found from the original list we came up with:

1. A Kasper suit in a rose color that fit her beautifully. The cut was traditional enough for her, and she noted that it would also go with some of her navy separates.

2. In women's, she found a cranberry pantsuit in a size sixteen that actually fit her, and she loved it. She announced when she came out of the fitting room that she wouldn't have cared if it was a size twenty-four—she loved it and it looked great on her!

3. She opted for a rose/brown blouse that looked lovely, and she also decided on a navy silk blouse with a brown paisley design on it. (This was to update her navy suit).

4. Two dresses, one was a typical traditional shift dress in baby blue. Rose was uncomfortable with anything sleeveless, so we found an off-white cardigan to go with it. Her old cardigan was too beat up to wear. (She pulled out a strand of real pearls for this dress ensemble.)

The other dress was a lightweight cotton in a light lemon and mauve pattern, with blue birds on it. Rose loved it and so it became her second summer dress.

5. We found one dress in a gabardine wool fabric at an outlet mall. It was an older style, but it was traditional enough that Rose could get many seasons of wear out of it. The dress was in a rich plum color, and she planned to wear a navy and plum scarf with it that she already owned. A pair of pearl earrings and she's out the door!

6. While she felt that her rose Kasper suit could stretch to a wedding, I nixed the idea. It was a little too deep in tone. However, I did point out a Kasper dress in soft pink. It wasn't one of her colors, so she waited. She later found a mint and mauve dress. It was lovely on her, and she went for that.

7. She found an off-white blazer that was on sale and worked perfectly with the pastels that were beginning to fill her closet. She also opted for a gray blazer and at last glance she had ordered a shorter jacket in powder blue.

8. She went crazy with slacks when she realized how good they looked on her. She bought five of the neutrals on her palette. The taupe and cocoa were so close she went for the taupe. The cocoa was an option for later on.

9. She bought a few bright-color T-shirts to go with her slacks for spring and summer. This was instead of the turtlenecks, because she decided to wait until next fall to see what the new colors brought.

10. She bought two polyester shells in yellow and watermelon. They were washable and made sense to her.

Rose found a job. She tells the story that she was wearing her rose-colored suit that was bought for the sole purpose of securing her future.

Over time, there were a few additions that she was to make to her daily wardrobe:

1. Skirts in her color family. (Rose did best in separates because she was one size larger on the bottom than on top.)

2. She was to subscribe to a few traditional catalogs such as Talbots.
3. She needed new undergarments.
4. Her shoes and other accessories needed updating; she agreed to set aside 10 percent of her paycheck for this.

Rose was off and running. Later she redid her home, too.

TRADITIONALS IN THE WORK FORCE

In some ways, Traditionals are as diverse in the work force as Trendys are. Although they are typically found in more conservative environments, Traditional women can operate as anything from housewife to president/CEO of a company.

And, if you happen to work with a Traditional, then you're in for a treat. She is never selfish and will do much more than is required of her. She's the one who will work through her lunch hour for her boss without complaining.

Who can ever forget "The Mary Tyler Moore Show" years ago? Even those in later generations get a sense of Mary's caring for her work "family." Mary made a nation of people accept that "work" family has as much value to some as the "home" family has to others.

Traditional women today redefine the role women play at home and in the workplace. In many ways they are the ones who are quite content to let the world be as it will, and go about their business. It's not that the Traditional woman doesn't care about the women's movement, it's just that she never felt that it was intended for her; she's never felt enslaved. She is and can be very strong and have powerful opinions of her own; yet she willingly takes a backseat on issues which she doesn't wish to undertake.

Ms. Traditional is a very busy woman and she picks and chooses her battles wisely. When environmental issues threatened her children's health, Meryl Streep spoke up about them.

When her husband was murdered, Coretta Scott King emerged as a leader, not because it was what she secretly desired, but because it was the proper role for her to take.

High profile Traditionals are as varied as first ladies Barbara Bush and Hillary Rodham Clinton. Eleanor Roosevelt was another powerful Traditional role model. While she never intended her life to be a political one, she, too, was drawn in by circumstances and didn't disappoint a nation.

Traditional women frequently undervalue their tremendous assets. Instead, they give as much as they can to those in their family.

Clothing?

It seems obvious that whatever she wears will reflect the more conservative of looks for whatever environment she is working in. Even Princess Diana, who may appear at times to be a Classic, never held the high ambition for herself that a Classic woman would. Traditional women have a gift for understatement and wear simple yet appropriate looks.

The Traditional woman's biggest obstacle in work circles is not in underselling herself, but in staying true to her style type. For while the flashy Dramatic may outshine her and the Classic may "outlabel" her, Traditional is always in style and always concerned for others in ways that her more "flashy" sisters may miss out on.

INTO YOUR CLOSET FOR SPECIAL OCCASIONS

1. White Tie—
Watch Angela Lansbury in any white-tie occasion on "Murder, She Wrote." Here is an example of timeless, traditional elegance. Also if you are looking for white tie, it should be easy to find something at a department store or specialty shop. Many stores carry a few looks for these kinds of traditional occasions, and as is the custom, you'll be able to find something perfectly you. Give yourself adequate time to locate a dress.

2. Black Tie—
I've never seen a Traditional who has missed wearing a long sheer skirt and sequin

blouse, or whatever kind of top is in at the moment. A satin blouse or charmeuse blouse in one of her personal colors can be sensational, too.

3. Black Tie Optional—

It is easy to get away with a wonderful day to evening dress. Just make sure not to underdress. When a Traditional woman underdresses, she can appear very inappropriately dressed.

Go for the *option!* Don't underdress for black tie optional. Even if you're sitting there reading this and thinking, "Well, I don't want to stand out," don't underestimate the powerful impression that your choice of attire can make upon others.

4. Cocktail Reception—

Pull out one of your lovely silk shift dresses (or even linen or wool). Fabric isn't quite as important here as effect. It's easy enough for you to go right from your office to a party with just a few simple accessory swaps. Add one or two strands of pearls to the one you already wear, perhaps even a pearl bracelet.

Leave the flat shoes in the car and endure an hour or two with heels, if you can. And, have fun!

Don't forget that for special occasions, choosing one of your personal colors will make mixing and matching easier. It also makes matching your existing shoes and handbags a snap.

To figure out what to buy for special occasions, consider this: Are there any colors on your collage that surprise you? Any styles? See if you can find them in the stores, but if you can't, consider having them made.

TOWN OR COUNTRY?

Angela Lansbury is a city Traditional. Over the years on her popular series, "Murder, She Wrote," the character of Jessica Fletcher slowly bloomed from a country Traditional, with her down-home charm, to a smoother city Traditional woman. I suspect that the actress herself needed to play someone more in tune with herself, especially over such a long time.

The preppie look years ago grew from the idea of taking a country traditional and transplanting it in the big city.

The wardrobe from country to city is surprisingly similar. For whether in the city or country, they are both Traditionals and will naturally be drawn to clothes appropriate for their life-style and environment.

TRADITIONAL WARDROBE BASICS

The idea of buying a new "outfit" is typically Traditional, and as you begin to think in terms of expanding your whole wardrobe and using what's in your closet, you'll create dozens of new combinations out of the clothing you already own.

There are some basic recommendations I make for Traditional women:

1. A haircut and style update
2. A print blouse to wear with neutral suits. Also a print skirt. If two-piece dressing seems appealing, ask yourself, "Can I wear this outfit three different ways?"
3. Pearls, if you don't have any. A few strands and some earrings, too.
4. A Coach handbag. (Or something similar. Buy good quality here.)
5. A weekend outfit that you can wear with your white Keds or Topsiders (that's sporty to you)! This can be borrowed from some of the beautiful Romantic dress styles available.
6. A subscription to a traditional catalog—Talbots, Carroll Reed, L. L. Bean, and Lands' End are just a few examples.
7. A dress (in the pink or peach family—whichever is better for you). This is a dress to wear to church, a *bris*, or a garden party. It seems that Traditionals always have oodles of events to go to.
8. A Traditional suit, any vendor can possibly fit here
9. Updated belts

Replace some of those well-loved items that are too well worn to still wear.

> **Tip:** Make an appointment to consult with a hairdresser before you go for a cut. I suggest making your consultation appointment on a separate day. This way if you don't feel 100 percent positive about this person cutting your hair, you leave yourself room to cancel and find someone else. Don't be polite and let someone cut your hair who you don't feel great about!
>
> **Tip:** Wear your real pearls often. Body oil is actually good for them. Store them in a breathable box or cloth; airtight places dry them out.

YOUR ACCENT STYLE

As a Traditional, you must always be sure that no matter what style you use as an accent, the focal point should always be Traditional. No one else looks as misplaced as a Traditional wearing the wrong style.

A TRADITIONAL TRAVELING

My friend Kayellen was good enough to give me her packing list. She is a pure Traditional, and these are her basics for travel. Since I had each style type make up their own list, this will vary in format from the other chapters.

Below is what Kayellen would pack for a five-day trip:

a) Khaki trousers
b) Jeans
c) One pair of khaki or navy walking shorts
d) Sneakers
e) One pair of low-heeled shoes that can go either with shorts, slacks, or skirt
f) Chambray skirt/blouse set
g) Navy blazer—single-breasted with navy buttons
h) White T-shirt-style top or mock turtleneck
h) Simple earrings (like a pair of small gold hoops)
i) Nylons, ankle socks for sneakers
j) leather-banded watch
k) thin leather belt

As you can see, basic, clean, and simple looks carry her for a few days!
The additions for business are:

a) Small pearl earrings, necklace
b) One full suit, and three blouses to wear with it
c) A short Chanel-style jacket (wool or cotton)
d) One dress to be worn with a blazer. Stay neutral or add one of her personal colors to the mix.
e) Two pairs of shoes, one low-heeled, one flat
f) One briefcase or tote bag, depending upon what is appropriate for your business

The additions for a trip to the Caribbean/Hawaii are:

a) One-piece bathing suit (Kayellen's is a navy blue Anne Cole)
b) One sundress with a dropped waistline can be worn with or without a T-shirt
c) One pair leather thong-style sandals
d) One pair of shades
e) A few headbands to keep hair off your neck and face.

Sporty

Comfort and flexibility within her style will highlight a Traditional with Sporty accents. A baseball cap or other fun piece looks adorable on a Traditional/Sporty. Don't go overboard, though, or you may wind up looking too out of place.

Romantic

Romantic mixes best with Traditional. Many Romantic silhouettes can work beautifully on a Traditional woman. It is important, however, that you only add a few silhouettes here and not go crazy. A beautiful floral dress with a 1940s traditional jacket can look very sharp indeed.

Shoes are a breeze since either romantic or traditional styles will do. A romantic accent could be a shoe with a bow, rather than a spectator pump. Why? Because spectators are typically best with hard traditional-fabric looks, while more femininely styled shoes will complement the movement in the flowing silhouettes of a romantic style.

A Traditional with a romantic accent can wear more floral looks than the average Traditional, and soft fabrics will work better on her. She'll love the ease of movement with her clothing. Remember though, Tradition reigns.

Traditional

Traditional accents are antique pins, old-fashioned brooches, scarves that are from another era, small purses, and anything that could be considered preppie. The preppie look is really a pure Traditional, who wears traditional accents.

Classic

Classic can be a confusing mix, and since Traditional and Classic are close, distinctions must be made. Classics will spend much more money on their clothes, preferring designer labels and silhouettes.

A Traditional woman should be wary of buying a designer suit that is too fashion forward for her. Traditionals tend to learn how to tie scarves and often use them, whether or not they are "in," while Classics will follow trends and wear only what's in. A very traditional accessory would be spectator pumps, while a Classic would only wear them if it was "in" that season.

My strong suggestions would be to proceed with caution here. Some of the most confusing looks result from women who unevenly blend these two styles. Be especially careful to stay traditional with belts, bags, and coats.

Dramatic

Grace Kelly is an example of a Traditional whose accent was Dramatic. Her home and family were put before all else, yet she was pulled into the spotlight throughout her life.

No matter what she wore, Grace Kelly wore it with dramatic accents. While her core was traditional, she accessorized with extreme elegance. Appearance and presence were very important to her. Only a Traditional/Dramatic would be that impeccable (and make a statement) all the time.

Trendy

Admittedly an odd mix, but surprisingly elegant. A Traditional/Trendy will mix and match her own touches into a traditional wardrobe beautifully. She will skim the magazines, decide which pieces she can use to update herself for a season, and—voila!—a new wardrobe. This woman is one fast shopper!

Simply by the nature of her talent for working with her wardrobe, she will move easily through thrift or department store in search of things that work for her.

She will lean toward accent items that are as individual as she is, since being herself within her family unit will be important to her.

COLOR WITH YOUR OWN PERSONAL STYLE

Every style type brings her own individual energy to a color. Traditional brings her respect for tradition to whatever color she chooses to wear, so keep that in mind when using the color glossary later in the book (Chapter Fourteen). Here is a brief synopsis of the basic colors and the Traditional woman.

A Red Outfit

This is almost a contradiction in terms. Dashes of red such as a stripe or an accessory are more appropriate for a Traditional woman. Wine, burgundy, or pink would be her choice, as they will give her the energy of red without the bold quality that doesn't quite fit her style.

A Traditional woman, unlike a Classic (Nancy Reagan), may not choose a suit in pure red. However, she may have a long flowing red dress that she wears with gobs of pearls to a fancy dinner party. By changing the silhouette—in this case a suit is replaced by a long flowing red dress—she can wear the color in her style without changing the impact of the color.

An Orange Outfit

A Traditional's natural warmth is heightened in orange. Whichever shade or hue of orange she wears will often reflect her current concerns for her family and loved ones.

A Yellow Outfit

When a Traditional woman wears yellow, it strengthens the color's cooperative message. Originality is not on her mind; for her, it is in old-fashioned tradition that lies great wisdom.

She'll wear yellow to lend cooperation and show her intentions as a team player.

A Green Outfit

In green, a Traditional woman finds a home for her nurturing and loving nature. Ms. Traditional connects with her passion for home and family when she dons green.

A Traditional woman will wear green anywhere and everywhere—from church to a wedding—for matters of the heart are her trademark.

A Blue Outfit

When she wears blue she expresses to others that not only is she trustworthy, but she trusts them, too. She always expresses the purest elements of blue—honesty and loyalty. Barbara Bush is a perfect example here. Can you remember her wearing anything *but* blue?

When she wears blue, Ms. Traditional conveys her fierce loyalty to those she loves (or works with) and expresses her unwavering loy-

alty and commitment. Be it on a weekend walk with the family or a meeting with the joint chiefs of staff, her sincerity is unwavering.

An Indigo Outfit

Independent indigo is a surprise on the Traditional woman, for it would tell others that she uses her intuition in her decisions. A Traditional woman, however, consults others too frequently to feel completely comfortable in indigo.

Now, I'm not saying that she doesn't trust her own instincts. Not so. She simply feels consulting those she loves and/or respects is vital when it comes to decision making.

A Purple Outfit

The royalty of purple is lost on a Traditional woman. She revels in the beauty of the color and appreciates its richness, but Ms. Traditional wears purple because she loves the elegance of it.

The idea of regal and royal colors worn to overpower others isn't her, for she could never feel comfortable pretending to be better than another person. The positive attributes of purple are heightened when Ms. Traditional wears it. Her natural grace adds to the spirituality of the color.

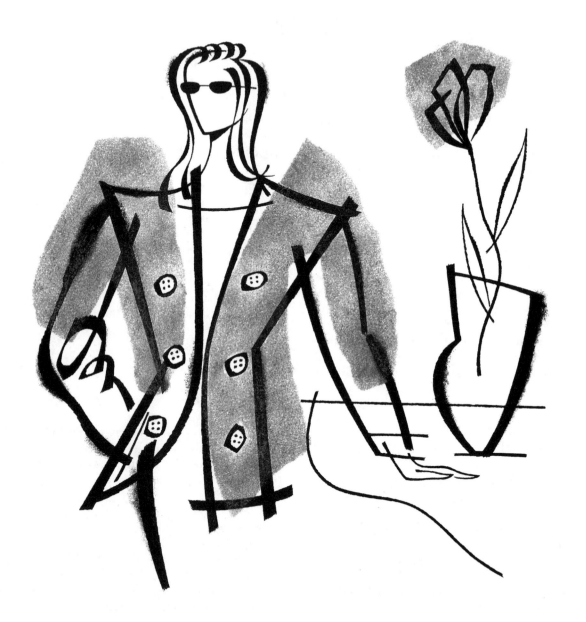

Chapter Seven

CLASSIC

Between Traditional and Dramatic is the Classic woman. This woman is never understated like a Traditional or overstated like a Dramatic. She frequently appears collected and almost always chooses the perfect business attire.

Absorbed by her work, she is the most overtly career driven of all the style types. This is inherent in her clothing purchases. This is the woman who knows the power of buying expensive, well-made clothing and enjoys wearing it. She buys top quality for herself and makes noticeable improvements in her man's wardrobe as well.

She does enjoy dressing her family and decorating a home. Her flair for style is matched only by her natural interest in it, which is why many Classics are recognized for their decorating talent.

Being a wife and mother can become a prominent career when undertaken by a Classic woman. Jacqueline Kennedy's life is a true testament to a Classic woman's complexity—

consider her passionate devotion to her family, her restoration and decoration of the White House, and in later life, her ability to find a career in publishing.

A Classic woman works for others, but never undersells herself. You'll find her in airports traveling with other business people, yet never dragging her luggage—she rarely overpacks. By nature, she is very good at organization and development.

Although she appears coordinated and almost perfect to the outside world, to those who know her well she is quirky. Classic's appear serious, but they can have a strange, almost wicked sense of humor.

She might not have gotten enough sleep, yet she's not a big complainer. This person is not only a trouper, she's completely dedicated to her work.

As a boss, she's wonderful! Fair and sincere, Classic's are warm and caring, often considering their employees before themselves. This quality surprises people because Ms. Classic seems so serious and self-absorbed. You'll be glad to be a part of her team, because she truly is a team player and will carry much more than her share of the load.

Department stores and finer specialty stores cater to Classics, however she'll have to watch those Dramatic personal shoppers, as they can put her in clothes that are too showy for her.

The Classic woman generally reaches for a designer label before a bargain brand. It's not because she's label conscious; she's quality conscious. This woman is a clotheshorse. If shopping were an Olympic sport, you can be sure that a Classic would nab the gold medal. Of all the style types, Classics could be considered the most trend conscious, since they stay abreast of what's happening. What they consider "bummy" is nice casual wear to many.

Ellen Tracy "is" Classic. Like the woman who wears the label, it is classically fashionable and never goes out of style.

RECOGNIZING A CLASSIC

Most of the famous Classics are so obviously classic, no matter what they do, they don't blend.

Classics tend to stand out. They are unable to disappear or take a backseat like a Traditional can. Meryl Streep, a Traditional, easily metamorphoses into another person. Jane Fonda, as remarkable a career as she's had, is unmistakably a Classic. In the roles she has portrayed, her personality has always been clearly there. In all the roles she played, Audrey Hepburn's personality was unmistakably present, too.

Many female newscasters are Classic, enjoying the limelight but needing it on their own terms. Connie Chung and Diane Sawyer are examples of high-profile Classic women in television news.

Candice Bergen as Murphy Brown and Phylicia Rashad as the mother on "The Cosby Show" are both examples of Classic women in television roles. Both of these women were perfectly matched to their roles.

What are the elements that make an outfit classic?

Quite often, Classic women ask me if it's now all right to wear blended fabrics. Their mothers (probably Traditionals) told them to only buy pure cotton or pure linen, never blends of any kind. Classics can and do wear blends and they often try new fabrics or combinations.

The real skill that a Classic possesses is the ability to build a wardrobe from pieces, unlike her Traditional sister who buys by the outfit. Unlike the streamlined simplicity of a Traditional, a Classic breaks the rules by mixing and matching to put together looks and create new twists.

The Classic's style is driven by her career, therefore you'll notice a business polish to even her most casual looks. This is the one element that delineates a pure Classic. Even in her off time, she's elegantly adorned and ready for business.

Skirt length is not an issue for a Classic woman; she can wear above or below the knee easily. She does tend to follow the flow of fashion, and if the tide is in she wears it short, if out, she wears it long.

Traditional looks can be worn beautifully by a Classic, but they don't quite fit. If you study the two styles you'll see that the timelessness of a Traditional doesn't quite fit the more contemporary Classic woman.

When I see good-quality knits with classic detailing (gold or silver buttons, or even crests when they're in style) I know it's perfect for a Classic. This look carries the natural elegance with it that Ms. Classic requires.

The key to nailing down a Classic, incidentally, is to simply rule out Traditional or Dramatic (or any other type, for that matter). The polish of an anorak could appear to be Sporty, but it is typically classic since it works with her more structured pieces, giving a casual look with an upscale feel.

Classic touches? Bold earrings (gold or silver) and matching chain belt (chain belts go in and out of style, so watch trends here). Look for polished button detailing and pieces that stand strong without being dramatic.

A CLASSIC STORY

One of my very first clients was a Classic. Andrea had grown up with a Dramatic mother, as had I, so we had hours of shared commiserating and laughter. She too had grown up with the belief that Classic meant boring.

CLOSET OR COLLAGE?

Since I worked with Andrea prior to my development of the collage approach, her statement was vital. She had told me in one of our first conversations that she had just bought the company she had been working for after an inheritance came through for her. In her statement, she expressed a desire to make the transition from employee to boss in her wardrobe.

Andrea's closet was a compilation of looks that had worked for her over the years, but as she outgrew or wore things out, she didn't replace them. She wound up mixing and matching pieces in her wardrobe, but was missing basic classic pieces that would create the focal points of her look.

I began by building on her strengths.

COLORS IN HER CLOSET

Once we hung her closet in color order, she began to see how her three personal colors were not only well represented, everything she owned worked with them in some way. She had instinctively not shopped into a dead end.

Her personal colors were:

1. Salmon was the color she felt best wearing (how she sees herself),
2. Light beige was the color she received the most compliments on (how the world sees her), and
3. Medium purple was the color she felt powerful wearing.

It was easy to see she was a "spring" coloration, and we easily located her colors on that wheel. Her personal colors also lent me insight into her personality.

I suggest you first look up the meanings in the color glossary (Chapter Fourteen) and see what they tell you about Andrea before reading my responses.

The salmon color represented who she really is inside. This told me that she is deeply spiritual. She holds her faith close to her heart and inspires countless others without even being aware of it. Believing strongly in equality, she isn't afraid to do whatever it takes to get the job done.

A neutral color liked beige seemed an odd color to receive compliments on, since this is also the way the world perceives you. Neutral. Interestingly, beige told me that Andrea is perceived by others as a woman who can produce results based on her steadfast manner.

And finally, purple as her power color tells me that her purpose stems from a belief that whatever she undertakes, she does for the highest good.

This is a woman who is career-minded, but spiritual about it. Her determination and focus were all about work (as can happen with a Classic), and we'd need to add a more casual, down-to-earth side to her wardrobe.

She had a small brown section in her closet, which she admitted she wanted to develop but didn't see the point since she owned so little of it. I disagreed; brown was a wonderful for her. I suggested she build it up, since it worked with all three of her personal colors.

THE SHOPPING LIST

Almost all her clothes were classic, and then I noticed almost all her jewelry was Trendy. It became clear that her accent was Trendy, so we left those pieces alone. Her wardrobe contained a beautiful array of pieces (remember that I'm a Classic, so this was heaven for me).

1. Anne Klein II
2. A-Line
3. Ellen Tracy
4. Dana Buchman
5. Some Liz Claiborne
6. Calvin Klein accents (leans toward trendy)

Keep in mind that there are literally dozens of other manufacturers that can and do make classic silhouettes. All of them change their focus from season to season. In any given month, they can create silhouettes for any style type, so don't go by vendors to judge your style, go by your quiz results.

In Andrea's case, I had to introduce her to a few catalogs that sold beautiful knits because we needed to relax some of her hard lines.

Two catalogs I added to her mailing list were Neiman Marcus by mail (800-825-8000), and Clifford and Wills (800-922-0114). Both of these catalogs carry a good supply of classic silhouettes.

There were a few things that we needed to add to Andrea's wardrobe;

1. A two-piece knit outfit. This was to begin a much-needed travel ensemble.
2. A two-piece suit that matched (could be pant and jacket)
3. A cocktail dress (a must for her new position)
4. A new suit in a neutral color
5. Basic blouses to match with her new suits and older separates
6. A few classic accessories to tone down her trendy accents. Being the new boss, she needed to make a strong statement. Nothing does this better than dressing in your own style from head to toe.

7. A watch (preferably gold)
8. A neutral shoe

THE RESULTS

There was more on her list than we first realized, and it took some time to locate what Andrea needed.

1. She ordered a light beige knit ensemble from Victoria's Secret. It was perfect for her.

2. We came across a smashing Dana Buchman suit in a medium purple that she fell in love with! She bought the jacket (which had a tie belt), the matching skirt, and I encouraged her to get the matching silk shell. I don't think tonal dressing is right for everyone, but it certainly looks magnificent on some Classics. Besides, medium purple is her power color.

On the same trip we came across an Ellen Tracy suit in salmon. She bought this suit with both a pant and a jacket. She would later come back and pick up the other key pieces to the group.

Both of these suits made sense for her. They were both perfectly classic and in her colors. It was a wise purchase.

As a Classic, the jackets are always the key piece. Make sure they are classic enough to wear season after season.

> **Tip:** Buy the key pieces of a collection when you see them. A blazer and skirt, for example. Come back later to pick up the other pieces when they go on sale. For a Classic it almost never makes sense to wait for an entire group to hit markdown since being current is part of her style. In addition, there are times when getting a full season's of wear out of your clothes is far more important than price.

3. She opted for a Donna Ricco dress for work that would double into evening for her. She fell in love with the cut and discovered a new vendor.

4. Another suit! This time it was a light gray Ellen Tracy that was exquisite. She opted for an off-white silk shell, and while this suit wasn't an important wardrobe builder, it served a valuable purpose.

She was having meetings where she was being forced into the role of arbitrator. Gray is the perfect color since it gives off the energy that the person wearing it is neutral in every way and doesn't take sides. The whole package worked.

5. Andrea located a stunning blush color cotton knit sweater from Calvin Klein, and it was perfect with her new purple suit.

She also came across a few silk and cotton blouses in buff, honey, and light beige.

6. We added a few Anne Klein II large faux earrings, Liz Claiborne, and Givenchy. While her trendy accents were fun (funky gold keys on a long key chain, for example), they just weren't the image that she needed to portray right now. It became apparent to her just how important her personal unity was. Her company had been through quite a bit in her takeover, and she wanted to convey a strong sense of cohesive leadership.

Part of this was achieved by simply creating solid head-to-toe classic ensembles. The other key to total congruence for a Classic is using your personal colors for a very powerful impact. Creating head-to-toe congruence is the only way to dress for optimal effectiveness.

7. She had been wearing a watch pendant, which was bordering on Dramatic and/or Trendy. We replaced it with an AKII gold chain watch. She had my word that she could still use her pendant for her weekend attire.

8. A flat gold shoe was her neutral shoe. It happened to be "in" when she bought it. Metallic shoes are fantastic for a Classic since they span her wardrobe. Don't make the mistake of wearing them if they're not "in" or you'll look like a dinosaur. Just put them aside, they'll be back in a season or two.

In addition, she did need to make a few additions to her daily wardrobe:

1. Play clothes. Cotton knit separates. She ordered the Allen Allen catalog (800-422-0466) from time to time; they have some great classic pieces.
2. Men's trouser-style pants, her pendant watch could be worn here
3. A denim workshirt (to go with the trousers)
4. Three oversized nice fleece sweatshirts to lounge in
5. A brown belt with a gold buckle, for her jeans

It was almost a year later that I developed the collage, and by then she had come back to work with me to update her wardrobe. This time I had her do the collage.

Her collage was very streamlined. All the outfits she wanted in her wardrobe were on her collage, and I made a few suggestions on where she might locate a few things and she was off and running.

Andrea called me a few months later and said she was going to do the collage once a year to update her wardrobe.

Unfortunately, I lost a client because she didn't need me anymore. But it was well worth it. It perfected my system. The collage provided the visual aid that I had been enlisted previously to do for the client.

Remember: It's primarily in the spring and fall where we really work at updating our wardrobe, because that's when the new styles are introduced.

A CLASSIC TRAVELING

Since I'm a Classic, I thought I'd give you my packing list. Here's what I usually bring with me to the Caribbean (I try and go at *least* once a year).

a) Underwear for the trip (a pair a day)

b) One pair of shorts, in khaki

c) T-shirt with a design or stripes. Never more than two. I usually buy a T-shirt.

d) Jeans, sometimes a color

e) A pair of nice pants. Linen, sometimes, usually a nice cotton

f) One cotton/lycra skirt to wear over bathing suits and under a T-shirt to shop or have an afternoon iced tea in. A pareo is a wonderful substitute, and since it's just a square yard of fabric, it doesn't take up a whole lot of room in a suitcase.

g) One blouse to go "out" in. Something nice to wear with my pants.

h) One pair each of sandals, beach thongs, and sneakers. I don't pack more than one pair of each. Shoes weigh a lot and chances are you won't wear them all anyway. Who cares about your feet? You're in the Caribbean!

i) Limited jewelry. Often I buy something on the trip, and there's no need for any "fine" jewelry.

j) One KMO—Knock Me Over—skirt (to pair with an equally devastatingly fine blouse) or an "easy" dress that is KMO

k) If you work out, bring a mini bag. One T-shirt, shorts, and socks. (If you prefer, leotards). They can all be rinsed out.

The colors I pack are black and white and I add one color. For me, it's indigo. This way, shoes are easy, white or black, and I simply throw a scarf or two into my suitcase, and I'm ready to go!

My variations for business are:

a) My Anne Klein jewelry in gold and silver

b) One full suit and three blouses for it (I can dry-clean on the road)

c) One "hot" skirt and blouse with a sweater to switch off from the suit

d) Two pairs of pumps, no sandals. In case I break a heel, I always have a backup.

e) Panty hose. Two pairs of every color I may need.

CLASSIC WARDROBE BASICS

1. A cocktail dress. Shop carefully here and take your time. Set aside some money to buy this. You'll have it for years, so this will be a small investment. Classics go to quite a few cocktail parties.
2. Another softer dress for day occasions, again take your time and invest here.
3. A KMO blouse (print if you'd like) to wear with linen pants, a classic belt, and Cole-Haan shoes. I've had an animal print blouse for over six years, when it's in I wear it, when it's out, it hangs in my closet. This is a good investment piece since it comes back every few seasons.
4. Assorted knits to wear for travel and not so "suited" times. Weekend wear that is comfortable, yet classic.
5. Hair ornaments in a variety of colors. Especially if you are a petite, you'll need to carry your color up—hair ornaments are great for that.
6. A new suit. I suggest adding a suit in a key color that you may be missing.
7. Weekend wear. Check out A-Line (Anne Klein) or Max Studio. While both of these labels can carry some trendier or dramatic items, there are a few beautiful classic pieces. Don't forget Calvin Klein!
8. Accessories are crucial to most Classics. You need earrings that will never go out of style. I also suggest adding a few basic watches. It is a classic accessory that if changed, doesn't usually scream "notice me," yet gives out the subtle message that you pay attention to detail.
9. A good pair of shoes is usually on my suggestion list. If flat shoes are needed, I suggest you add a neutral color here.
10. Belts? You have to review them. Basics here; black with gold buckle for work, black with silver for jeans. You may need a white (or colored) belt as well.
11. I might also put either a pair of black or white jeans on your list. Perhaps a color, if you wish.
12. A pair of trouser pants—Classics look very elegant in menswear. Different elements of it come and go, but a good khaki trouser for casual wear is a must.

Hardest to find for a Classic? A good jogging suit or pair of sweats. I recommend adding this, too.

CLASSICS IN THE WORK FORCE

Ms. Classic is all business! This is a woman who takes her career seriously. Sometimes to the exclusion of all else. Balance is often a problem for a Classic woman because she cares so much—correction, *too* much—for her work.

Classic women make great lawyers, doctors, and top executives because they are cool under fire. They naturally have a stronger constitution, which enables them to surmount obstacles that would stop others.

There is a courageousness to Ms. Classic, and a seriousness that her inner dedication only intensifies.

She can work long hours focusing intense concentration on her work. She is a wonderful worker, but not always the best employee. Her natural need to excel will be not out of a lust for power, but from a realization that she's mastered this and is ready to move on.

Frequently overqualified, she can find herself frustrated in any situation where she is not running the show. Unlike others, Ms. Classic frequently needs to break out on her own and try new things.

Her driving ambition is just a part of the Classic makeup. Her drive for excellence shows in everything she does—her career, relationships, and life. And of course, her wardrobe.

Look for Ms. Classic doing anything that requires giving more than is humanly possible. She will desire to reach higher and do better constantly. Success is a given with a Classic woman.

Oh, incidentally, she will approach family with the same intensity as her career. So her children's teachers will definitely know her!

Her choices for career clothing will be the absolute best available for her. A Classic probably coined the phrase "Less is more." She won't need much, but she will require good quality.

INTO YOUR CLOSET FOR SPECIAL OCCASIONS

1. White Tie—

Here you can take your lead from a few former first ladies. Pick up a few old *Life* magazines and look at Jacqueline Kennedy's ball gowns or Nancy Reagan's. Yes, they will be outdated. But you will see some Classic styling ideas. And perhaps even create a gown that works for you.

Remember, Classic is a sophisticated elegance. Never understated, never flashy. Always appropriate.

2. Black Tie—

This is a natural for a Classic woman since she lives her life as if it's a black tie event.

In your closet there are probably a few separates already waiting for you. Silk or satin pants with a sequined top. A sheer skirt with a sexy blouse in a fabric, or some little jacket with sequins, that spells evening.

Buying a dress is an option, too. Consider how frequently you'll wear it, however. Romantic Marilyn Monroe wore a tight-fitting white dress and looked smashing, but you'll require a silhouette and design that flatters but doesn't advertise. Think of your style before you buy that sexy little sequin number.

3. Black Tie Optional—

Finally, I can't tell you how much this type of invitation annoys me.

There you are, all ready for action, wearing a beautiful dress appropriate for black tie, and your date shows up wearing a suit. Sorry. As a Classic woman that drives me crazy! Coordinate with whoever you're going with. Find out what the host/hostess is really wearing.

> **Classic rule:** Never outdress the person throwing the party.

Wear black tie unless you can't due to a previous business meeting, etc.

4. Cocktail Reception—

For you? Practically anything in your closet. Any of your better suits would work, or even your dresses.

TOWN OR COUNTRY?

A Classic in a country environment would still be focused on career. A country Classic dresses as impeccably as a city Classic.

So there really is very little difference.

In fact, a Classic is basically a city personality; she's high-powered and constantly on the go. Classics tend to stand out in the country, not quite blending in with their environment. They can easily be thought to be dramatic since they don't quite fit in.

Don't misunderstand. Classics can and do live in the country, they are just better suited to city life.

YOUR ACCENT STYLE

Since you already possess a natural flair for style no matter where you are, it's consistency that can be your big hang-up. Let's take a look at how each accent affects you. In addition to this, I suggest reading the chapter on your accent style.

Sporty

Anything fun and new will find its way into your wardrobe if you possess sporty accents.

Except they will be of the finest quality. For example, if whistles on a chain are all the rage, you will own it in the finest silver or gold-plated; always the best costume jewelry you can find.

In addition, you will tend to choose an elegant ski suit if you are a skier (for example). If Sporty is your accent, functional Classic clothes are important to you. Classics who live in the country tend to have more functional sporty clothes that work with their environment.

Romantic

A Romantic accent for you may include a short feminine jacket, as well as some beautiful lace tops. Romantic fabrics that move and feel elegant will find their way into your wardrobe. Your ability to mix these accent pieces in with your style can make you appear trendy. Be sparing with your romantic pieces and make sure you maintain your classic edge in everything, otherwise you will dilute your wardrobe and confuse others.

Traditional

A Classic whose accents are traditional will always be dressed impeccably no matter how sloppy she feels. While her career is important to her, it is her family that her career decisions will be wrapped around.

The addition to her accessories will be pearls, which she probably already has. Also, scarves tend to be big in the wardrobe of a Classic with traditional accents, as do tiny purses.

Classic

DKNY belts, Chanel accessories (some), AKII jewelry, Givenchy jewelry. High-quality shoes—Cole-Haan, Charles Jourdan, and Amalfi all carry a variety of style types, but there are quite a few beautiful Classics in there, too.

Dramatic

Bold earrings and fabulous accessories are part of this accent. This woman is extremely career driven and excels in whatever she undertakes. But humility about her accomplishments is a classic trait. They are more real than a pure Dramatic, who often takes on a fairy-tale quality in the media. A Classic/Dramatic is driven and stubborn, but always has a graciousness to her style that makes her accessible and desirable to the public.

She will accessorize to draw attention, but never outlandishly. Always Classic.

Trendy

The ever-important key to this blend is to remember that each piece should stand on its own, and no more than one trendy or unusual item as an accent, otherwise you may run the risk of looking like something out of a thrift store. Pay special attention to staying with classic looks, but *do, do, do* experiment with fabric mixes and shoes. Have fun, this is a daring combination!

COLOR WITH YOUR OWN PERSONAL STYLE

A Classic brings a professional touch to whatever color she is wearing. Her impact on others is career related.

A Red Outfit

There was a time when a red suit would have been pretentious to wear to work; times have changed. A Classic woman in red adds an air of elegance to an otherwise outspoken color. She states that she is not afraid to let her opinion be heard, but she finds it unnecessary. She commands attention just through her presence and others respect her as the woman in charge.

A Classic woman may wear red to a client lunch or to a meeting with her new employees.

An Orange Outfit

"Follow my lead" is the inspired message that Ms. Classic sends out when wearing orange. She leads the way by beginning the task at hand and soon others are following her. The active energy of orange inspires movement.

When Ms. Classic dons orange during her leisure time, it is to draw from the warmth of orange and relax. A Classic will often have some shade or hue of orange (ie. coral) in her home as well, for a feeling of warmth is very important to her.

A Yellow Outfit

Ms. Classic in yellow? Take charge. She is giving a message that she is precise—as is her nature—and intelligent.

In yellow weekend wear she is the perfect match for the "planner" that she secretly is. She'll deny it, claiming that she's just as disorganized as the next person. Not so; in fact, she appears even more organized when she shows up wearing yellow.

A Green Outfit

The strong sense of balance created by a Classic when she wears green is not only felt by her, but by those around her. An aura of heartfelt kindness and generosity finds its home here. She also creates confidence in herself and others when wearing green.

Ms. Classic reaches for green when she feels the need to gain emotional understanding in a particular situation. If she seeks reconciliation or needs to express her feelings, green is the perfect choice for her. Since this is naturally her color, it is a wonderful harmonious choice for a Classic.

A Blue Outfit

One of the principal traits of Ms. Classic is her ability to communicate with others, and she may wear almost any shade of blue. As a Classic she is never out of style and when she wears blue, she tells others that her ideas are also current.

With blue, she highlights all elements of her spirituality and faith. She is communicating to others that she trusts and is loyal to them.

Whether a sky blue windbreaker to go sailing or a navy suit to a conference, blue is an integral part of a Classic's wardrobe because she understands the importance of communication.

An Indigo Outfit

Being confident and able to make on-the-spot decisions is what Ms. Classic assures others of when *she* dons indigo. For her, the color indigo can symbolize higher ideas being incorporated into everyday living.

She can carry the energy of indigo from boardroom to bedroom, for her instinct connects her to her business associates as well as loved ones.

Indigo can be a very powerful business ally for a Classic woman because it conveys to others that she is able to solve problems creatively. In indigo she is the perfect image of the self-assured woman who trusts her own instinct implicitly—and so will others.

A Purple Outfit

Respect for the imagination is Ms. Classic's strongest message in purple. This is a wonderful color for her to wear when she wishes to distinguish herself as being creatively imaginative.

She herself is already well respected, and the match with purple will only heighten that. Ms. Classic will distinguish herself from the rest of the pack when she wears purple.

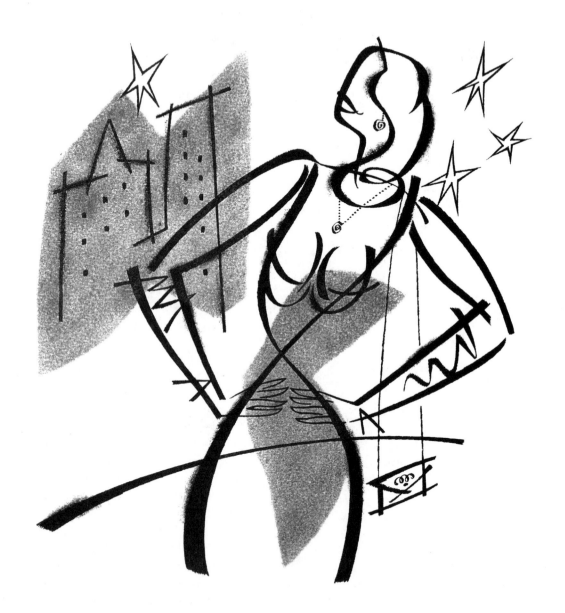

Chapter Eight

DRAMATIC

> **Famous Dramatics:**
> Joan Crawford, Joan Collins, Bette Davis, Elizabeth Taylor, Diana Ross, Anjelica Huston
>
> **Dramatic Focus:**
> Glamour
>
> **Dramatic Quote:**
> "If you produce results, then you are controversial; if you are mediocre, no one notices."

A Dramatic woman is aloof, independent, fiercely caring, and almost always in the limelight. From secretary to star, she can be found anywhere. She is striking, with a powerful presence that can only be compared to royalty. Ms. Dramatic is just as comfortable having tea with the Pope as she is at lunch with her closest friend.

This woman never simply enters a room, she makes an entrance, creating a stir wherever she goes. She is slightly outrageous, but her gutsy presence dares you to challenge her. Her flamboyant, outspoken manner may offend some. Dramatics can alienate others by being too demanding, for it's hard for her to accept that others are not always at their best the way she is (or appears to be).

She's the "Auntie Mame" type. Her choices are always daring, and surprising to many. She may stay single by choice, or if she marries, she may choose not to have children.

If she does have children, she will have to work hard at allowing them to develop without her domineering hand. If they rebel, and they will, she can be left feeling deeply wounded by their behavior when it is only what children do.

Ms. D may have a hard time being anything but right, and this makes for a tough relationship with a mate. Unfortunately, even though she is out of the spotlight when she arrives at home, she sometimes commands the same idolatry from her loved ones that she wants from strangers. This is not something that she does intentionally. Dramatics are naturally "on."

The important thing to remember is that a Dramatic, seemingly insensitive, really is as fragile as a lamb. Underneath her flair for the grand is really a woman who is sensitive and caring, perhaps even shy.

On the up side, Dramatics are not afraid to step up and make their presence known. I have yet to meet a Dramatic who can enter the room without causing a stir. Her instinct to wear what feels right for her is almost always right on. In my work with Dramatic women, the greatest challenge is in implementing a wardrobe of casual wear that she can live in.

Dramatic's know how to choose colors effectively. Bold, dramatic colors are worn well by Ms. Dramatic. It is almost uncanny how naturally a Dramatic woman will choose colors that tend to convey her strengths and downplay her weaknesses.

Ms. Dramatic's life-style is almost always centered around a city. If not, she may live removed from the public eye because she gets enough of it. She cannot stay away from adoring fans or admirers for a long period of time, however, or she begins to get grouchy, for it is in being noticed by others that Ms. Dramatic shines.

Bold dynamic styling makes the Dramatic woman come to life. Whether she chooses to wear pants with wide legs, tapered or tailored legs, leggings, or stirrups, it won't matter to her. What does matter is the colors she picks and the packaging she chooses to present her powerful message.

Clothing with severe lines and colors best demonstrates the image of the Dramatic woman.

RECOGNIZING A DRAMATIC

Elizabeth Taylor as Cleopatra was one of the more famous Dramatic matches. Angelica Huston in *The Addams Family* brought life and excitement to the role of Morticia Addams. A perfect match of Dramatic to Dramatic. Angelica Huston consistently matches her Dramatic personality to the right roles.

The forcefulness of Bette Davis was always a Dramatic. Even in her later life, she matched herself to her roles. When she was old enough to be a character actress, she took out an ad in *Variety* stating that a character actress was seeking work. This stunned the film industry, which had laid her to rest in their minds. The glamour of youth gone, there was nothing left.

Not so; Dramatics are not afraid to take a stand if they have to. In fact, when they truly don't care what others think, they can be majestic. Bette Davis had a remarkable career comeback later in life, filled with dignity and the public's respect.

Diana Ross is a Dramatic with a romantic accent. Her famous roles in *Lady Sings the Blues* and *Mahogany* were both Dramatic/Romantic and Romantic/Dramatic respectively.

How about a pure Dramatic? Joan Crawford. In any role she played, no matter how bad the movie was (and some were), she played a Dramatic. Here is a case where the actress became big despite the fact that she was labeled box-office poison. This is because she matched every role she portrayed.

When an accent and a style type match in a movie role like that, it often becomes a very memorable part for the actress.

Dramatics do tend to be movie stars rather than television stars, however. Joan Collins as Alexis Carrington on the television series "Dynasty" was an exception. Interestingly, Dramatic's on television enjoyed a burst of popularity in the 1980s. But Dramatics on television are rare. They are more popular on the big screen rather than television. Why? They're larger than life.

What are the elements that make an outfit dramatic?

The key to dressing for a Dramatic woman is that the focal point of her outfit must be *Dramatic*.

Almost anything she puts on will turn into an elegant affair. Even simple styles that may not appear to be much on others can be breathtaking on her. She knows the impact of her style and isn't afraid of overdoing it. Dramatics are always high fashion, no exceptions. This style is all about its magnified details.

Heavy accessories? A fabulous dramatic trait that only *she* can pull off. Attitude is important to a dramatic look; it's not always what she wears, but *how* she wears her clothes. This woman is mature.

Don't forget: Dramatics always use stand-out detailing.

Everything a Dramatic woman does is sexy and has tons of presence about it. Even a simple swimsuit could have a very sheer top. Sexy sarongs or sheer coverups are most definitely dramatic touches.

While other style types might wear certain things for a "special" occasion, Ms. D could wear it daily. Only a Dramatic woman can go to work in a suit that looks like she's stepping out to a cocktail party.

A DRAMATIC STORY

I did not know what to make of seventeen-year-old Gwendolyn. After she took the quiz, I was not surprised to discover that she was a Dramatic. At first I thought she was a Trendy, because she came to see me wearing a pair of ripped jeans, a large Ellen Tracy olive-colored belt that held up her pants (too wide for the loops, it was wrapped around her waist), matching olive shoes and suede shirt, leather jacket, and a black Russian-style hat. She walked in carrying a pair of red leather gloves.

It wasn't hard for me to see why her Traditional mother sent her to me, informing me, "She's all over the place. Maybe you can do something with her." Once I ascertained that Gwendolyn was a Dramatic, I knew Mom would not be thrilled if I worked on developing Gwendolyn's style further.

CLOSET OR COLLAGE?

When she brought her collage to me, I was stumped.

Her collage was filled with some of the most powerful natural images one could imagine. Thunderstorms with lightning descending from clouds and sunsets so vibrant they appeared painted on the sky, a volcano erupting, and images of fires and destruction. It could appear (to a parent in particular) that this young woman was obsessed with the tragic side of life.

As I sat with it and studied her work, I began to grasp what she was trying to say.

She saw the bold, dramatic side of life. This was not a game to her. She was aware of the truth in the world, but in that, she also saw what was naturally beautiful. She just perceived things in a very dramatic way.

Gwendolyn's collage revealed a more emotional nature, and she often confessed that she functioned best when she was in touch with nature. It was no surprise to discover that she was a bit of a daredevil, and on her eighteenth birthday went bungie jumping and made a plan to ride the rapids in the Grand Canyon the next year. Her choices for fun were dramatic, and they showed up in her collage. She was definitely a country Dramatic, since the outdoors and nature dominated her collage.

Gwendolyn didn't want to write a statement. She said she didn't understand what I was looking for. I told her that all she had to do was tell me who she was. I made it easier for her by giving her a list of famous people and telling her to write down whom she admired and why. Since she was dragging her feet on this, I told her to write it to me as a letter. This is an edited copy of her letter:

Dear Ms. Hartman,

When you said to me that I should think of people that I admire, I checked out the list you gave me and Grace Jones was the first person. She's always in control, like no one could get her. She is protected by her own power. I want to make a difference, but a lot of times I don't know how since I'm only one person. I don't get how this is going to help me with my style. My mom says I'm too wild and I need to tone down and act my age, but I'm confused. I don't know how to be like she tells me to be.

I like clothes and shopping. I like that people notice me. My friends always want to dress like me. Sometimes it bothers me that my mom wants me to be more like her. I love jazz and going out at night especially. I like being ultrafeminine, and I want jewelry that looks real; I hate fake-looking stuff. I don't care if it's expensive, just that it works the best on me.

Gwendolyn

Her statement did show growing pains, she was only seventeen at the time, but it was also quite clear that she was a Dramatic.

What were the clues to her being a Dramatic? Aside from the dramatic collage, there were several clues in her statement/letter. She said she wanted to be "ultrafeminine," and she also didn't care if she wore real jewelry, as long as it appeared to be real. She wanted her clothes to make a statement. These three clues gave me the idea she was a Dramatic. Why not a Trendy? Because Trendys never consistently care (across the board, the way a Dramatic will) about how others perceive them. A Dramatic is always concerned about making a powerful statement when she enters a room. Interestingly, her heroine was Grace Jones, a Trendy!

In Gwendolyn's case, the biggest job I had was convincing her mother that her child was fine. She was a Dramatic, and therefore needed to be allowed to develop her style and ideas apart from her mother.

Her wardrobe was one of a typical seventeen-year-old. And while I can tell you that she was anything but typical herself, her wardrobe was fairly standard. Gwendolyn was headed for a prestigious women's college in the fall, and her mother felt that her daughter needed a "new" wardrobe. She didn't.

About 75 percent of her wardrobe was made up of versatile, wearable clothes that were great choices for her. Most Dramatics already buy what they love.

COLORS IN HER CLOSET

Gwendolyn was young, and while teenagers do experiment, Dramatic's tend to be surprisingly consistent.

It wasn't hard to see Gwendolyn's three colors in her wardrobe. They were olive, red, and black. In a few minutes we had the lineup:

1. Olive was the color she felt best wearing (how she sees herself),
2. Red was the color she received the most compliments on (how the world sees her), and
3. Black was the color she felt powerful wearing.

As with many Dramatics, color charts didn't really influence her. I told her she looked like a winter and she responded that she was in her fall color phase.

She was right. Although the color she received the most compliments on was a true red, which is a winter color. And her power color, black, is also on the winter wheel.

Many women choose black as their power color, so this is not necessarily a good indication of the wheel to choose.

But it was olive, a color that belongs to the autumn chart, that she was most in tune with now.

Each of these colors gave me a powerful insight into this young woman. Before you read how I interpreted her colors, take a quick peek in the glossary (Chapter Fourteen) and see what the color definitions are for Gwendolyn's colors.

See what your conclusions are about her before you read mine.

Understanding a client through color always helps me to guide her more effectively toward appropriate clothing choices. The more in tune I can become with a client, her quirks, likes, and dislikes, the more able I am to guide her toward total congruence.

Let's start with Gwendolyn's olive.

This color choice tells me that Gwendolyn feels particularly solid in herself and strong in her convictions. She is open, and I suspect, feels a need to convey to her mother that she is trustworthy. Consistency is important to her, and she is deeply committed to it. For now.

True red is the color that she receives the most compliments in and also the way the world sees her. It was no surprise that she was a fireball, igniting ideas and getting things going by her sheer force of will. While she is a great starter, she's not much on follow-through. (Although the Olive counterbalances that.)

And finally, black tells me that she feels a deep need to be taken seriously.

So while Gwendolyn may not normally finish things, there's quite a bit at stake here for her. She has a strong desire to be taken seriously and is willing to make a commitment.

THE SHOPPING LIST

Gwendolyn's wardrobe was 75 percent there, a high percentage for someone so young, but not unusual for a Dramatic. I recommended some basics to fill in space since she was going to college in the fall (this was a cooler climate).

1. Three turtlenecks
2. Three pairs of jeans
3. Three sweaters
4. Two dresses
5. One funky fun standout piece that goes with the bulk of her wardrobe
6. One pair functional boots

Aside from this, she could bring her choice of jewelry, scarves, belts, hats, and any other accessories she felt she needed. In addition, she was going to bring along quite a few other pieces of clothing she already owned.

THE RESULTS

I know that her list doesn't appear dramatic in any way. I kept it simple on purpose. I knew no matter what we came up with she'd change it, which is typically a dramatic thing to do. I felt if I gave her a list of basics, she'd improvise and make them work for her.

Let's take a look at what Dramatic Gwendolyn came back with.

1. I suggested three turtlenecks; she bought: a royal blue sleeveless cotton turtleneck (she got one in black, too), a red henley-style sweatshirt, a white angora boatneck sweater.

2. I suggested three pairs of jeans, she bought: a long black sarong skirt in cotton, a short denim sarong, a pair of elegant wide-leg polyester pants in black.

3. I suggested three sweaters; she came back with: her father's college sweater in her true red, a sexy angora sweater in black, a long black cardigan in a silk knit.

4. I suggested two dresses; she bought: one long dress in black, one sheer dress in black and white.

5. I suggested one funky piece; she bought: one catsuit (her choice) in a bright multicolored design.

6. Sexy high-heeled black boots

She also bought some heavy black tights to wear with her short skirts and boots, as well as her torn jeans.

I wouldn't be telling you the truth if I

didn't admit that Gwendolyn's mother was disappointed by the job I did. She wanted me to turn her Dramatic daughter into a Traditional. I had failed. Gwendolyn, with all her talent and energy, needed to be supported in what her own instinct told her. A Dramatic's thinking is frequently ahead of her time, and rather than spend time trying to suppress that, I feel it's important to recognize and support it.

You may wonder why I chose someone so young as an example here. Two reasons: one, style problems aren't an age issue (or a size issue, for that matter), and second, of all the style types, a Dramatic's style develops the fastest.

Incidentally, there were a few additions to her daily wardrobe:

1. We stumbled across a DKNY blazer in icy pink that was sensational on her.
2. She was into sarong skirts, and I suggested two more: one in a red-and-black silk that would work with her henley or sleeveless turtleneck, and the other in white to go with her new blazer. Both skirts were three inches above the knee.

So let's now go to your closet and check for a few basics that as a Dramatic you'll want to be sure you have. If not, you can add them over time. Don't worry, your style won't change.

DRAMATICS IN THE WORK FORCE

At work, she knows just how to shine, and most likely what to wear. Dramatics don't always have the same ability with people, however. Her difficulty is not with employees, because she can communicate what she expects from them quite well; it's being a co-worker, not the boss, that she may have difficulty with. Even if she doesn't mean them to, others look up to her and can be intimidated by her presence.

Unlike the other style types, a Dramatic may need to tone down and blend. Not all the time, for that would go against her nature. However, that may be something she needs to do from time to time.

If you are a Dramatic, any company that has you as an employee is lucky. For presentations, dinners, or parties, you know how to present yourself well. Others seek out your guidance, and it is often you who runs the office, even if you're not the boss. Overly efficient, others look up to you as a leader, sometimes more than you are aware of. They admire your style, the way you handle difficult situations, and the way you speak up for yourself and others.

Others who work with you rarely have to take an assertiveness course; just being around you is a lesson in itself.

Success flocks to you, whether or not you want it. Even when you are lazy, opportunities are offered you that others would jump at. Once in the limelight, you rarely leave it.

INTO YOUR CLOSET FOR SPECIAL OCCASIONS

They haven't invented an occasion for which a Dramatic wasn't prepared. I frequently call my Dramatic friend Carolyn to get suggestions about what to wear to various events. She always knows. Her ability to throw together a fabulous look out of very little is only one tiny facet of her style.

Your biggest job will be to go through your closet and make sure that you have no out-of-date outfits that are simply not you. And to update constantly. But, for a Dramatic, that is not hard!

The truth is, most Dramatics I know have a closet full of clothes that they wear. There are very few mistakes in a Dramatic's wardrobe, at least few that I know they will admit to.

1. White Tie—
There is nothing more formal than a Dramatic woman in white tie. The greatest thing about this type of event for you is that you can rent a video or some period movie where the stars wore ball gowns and get ideas. Look for Joan Crawford or Bette Davis movies. The key to this look will be your own dramatic touches. Gloves and a hat will be two important elements of creating a dramatic white-tie look.

2. Black Tie—
For you, dressy wear in your closet would probably work for black tie. There isn't a Dramatic I know who isn't well equipped in this area.

I saw a Dramatic woman wearing a short black miniskirt, opera-length black gloves, and a sequined top. She looked sensational.

Long skirts and silk blouses are standards as well.

3. Black Tie Optional—
Ah, casual wear to you! But more than likely, you'll wear black tie, because black tie, optional or not, is formal to you.

Here you can get away with an elegant pair of pants or one of your elegant skirts and an exquisite blouse.

4. Cocktail Reception—
This is a natural for you. Sexy, powerful looks in vibrant colors or bold patterns. Nothing too demure for you, Ms. Dramatic.

I'm positive that it was a Dramatic woman who either invented or inspired shoulder pads, creating that powerful, hard look, that Joan Collins sported in the series "Dynasty" or the strong suits that Joan Crawford made famous.

TOWN OR COUNTRY?

Remember the show "Green Acres"? Eva Gabor was the perfect Dramatic. Living in the country, craving the city, longing for the place where she could lead the elegant life she loved.

And, conversely, the city Dramatic may crave the tranquility of the country. No matter where she is or where she wants to be, Ms. D will be dramatic about it.

Dramatics are by nature city girls. Many live or have lived in the country, but regardless, they tend to live in both worlds: one quiet and contemplative and the other loud and visible.

In a city Dramatic's collage, much more fashion and style will emerge. Armani suits may show up, and while other elements of her life may appear, they will all be bold and dramatic, and, interestingly enough, city activities will dominate.

In a country collage, dramatic images of tranquility may appear, or pictures of her version of "country" clothing. DKNY jeans and a workshirt, for example.

A DRAMATIC TRAVELING

I asked my Dramatic friend Lauren to put together her packing list for me. When I asked her for a business trip as well as a pleasure trip, she told me that she'd pack the same for both. Here is her list for a five-day trip:

a) Brown skin-tight Agnes B skirt with a slit up the front
b) Tight black cashmere sweater
c) One black sleeveless Danskin leotard (shiny material, they no longer make it)

d) Cream-colored crocheted short-sleeved tight shirt (She keeps her option for sexy or conservative with suiting)
e) 1950s dove gray cardigan
f) Cream-colored raw silk sweater
g) White denim Levi's

(continued)

h) two pairs funky genuine 1940s shorts: one beat-up drawstring khaki, one silk cream-colored shorts
i) Black bustier
j) Floor-length black chiffon dress, with matching short-sleeve duster
k) Kilim carpet mules
l) White low-top Converse All-Stars
m) Black platforms with ankle straps
n) Secretary-looking brown pumps ("If your shoes are out of date, it doesn't happen. I make sure mine are current.")
o) two pairs nude stockings
p) two pairs black stockings

q) two sexy black teddies
r) two sexy bras
s) two sexy panties (She rarely ever wears these since she wears bodysuits and panty hose.)
t) Ysatis by Givenchy
u) Chanel sunblock
v) Cocoa butter for her skin
w) Facial products
x) Her Oliver Peoples sunglasses and prescription glasses, also her contacts
y) Books
z) Diamond-stud earrings
aa) Garnet rings

Business additions:

a) Light wool Agnes B suit in dove gray, low cut (Jacket is shirtwaist style.)
b) A black low teddy for underneath (Evening and day double up here.)

c) Black or cream leotard for business

Options:

a) Pure silk Chinese shirt that has no buttons. She tucks it in criss-cross and wears a sexy teddy underneath.
b) A baby blue cashmere long-sleeved turtleneck sweater for wear over either Agnes B skirt

c) 1940s polka-dot dress in blue

The key to Lauren's wardrobe was mixing really expensive new pieces with inexpensive thrift-store items. She rarely wears cotton or linen, preferring her rich fabrics of cashmere, silk, or chiffon.

DRAMATIC WARDROBE BASICS

The first thing we consider are the three colors that you chose from your fashion color profile. These colors are probably dominant in your wardrobe as well. While most women do own a lot of black, probably you and Trendy share this as one of your frequently chosen personal "colors."

Unlike any other style type, color runs the show for you, since you are driven by high energy, and color conveys that to others.

Your three personal colors will encompass the three facets of your personality, and you can use each color to build your wardrobe with. Preferably, you should have an ensemble from each category of color that works for you.

Let's take the color that makes you feel the best to wear. Hanging in your closet should be clothes that you can wear when you feel

relaxed and close to those around you. As a Dramatic, you will be choosy as to who gets close to you, so this outfit should not be worn to a large banquet. This is the outfit to choose for social occasions where the groups are small and personal. A small garden party given by a close friend is a wonderful place to wear this ensemble. Or a walk on the beach with a loved one. For you, this is also the wonderful color to wear on a romantic date, where you want someone to get to know you. This category is weekend or casual wear to most women, and can be the most difficult for you. For these outfits, you may have to shop a bit, for this may not be hanging in your closet already.

At the minimum, this category (the color you feel best wearing) should contain:

1. A dress, for weekend
2. A soft sweater and pant
3. A casual ensemble

Keep in mind that this may be the hardest category for you to expand on. Because for you to feel good in something, it has to make a splash.

Second, let's look at the color that you receive the most compliments on. Incidentally, when you go to your closet in search of outfits in this category, you should find quite a few here. For being the hedonistic creature you are, praise is high on your priority list, and the bulk of your wardrobe will probably rest here. With that in mind, make a list of all the outfits you have in your most complimented color, then we will work at incorporating that color somewhere in your daily costume.

I suggest you have these items, whether or not you choose your complimentary color for them:

1. A silk print blouse to wear with your leather skirt or pant
2. An accessory so fabulous that they'll be talking about it for years
3. A hair ornament that makes a statement. A simple hair clip would never do for you, it must be a Wow! A fantabulous hat, bow, or string of bows. Whatever it is, it must be dramatic.
4. A pair of leather gloves that are as outspoken as you are. This is a good addition to any Dramatic's wardrobe. A colorful leather glove for cold weather or unlined for warmer climates and/or a pair of opera-length gloves for formal wear.
5. Dramatic Accessories. A bold pair of earrings, necklace, bracelet, etc. Bold chunky bracelets (or a few that make noise together) are great for a Dramatic; they draw attention each time you gesture. This can be in your most complimented color or just go well with it.
6. Panty hose is a critical purchase for a Dramatic. You need to have whatever the hose of the season is, patterned or not, and it should to match the things you wear. You can and do wear various prints and brands.
7. Belts are not as critical here, since you probably already have several phenomenal belts; however, check their condition, they may need replacing. If you need a new belt, buy one, but keep in mind that you may want any new purchases to work with your personal colors (in some way, contrasting is okay for you).
8. The shoe of the season
9. A pair of silk or gabardine pants. Then check your silk blouses to see if you need a new one.
10. A coat that makes an entrance. Long leather in a color, a plush (if they're in), a fur (fake if you prefer). Whatever it is, consider buying it in your most complimented or your power color.

And, finally, there's your power color. Unlike any other style type, this will be a full category because you pull energy from this color.

A few things you may want to find here:

1. A suit
2. Accessories
3. A fabulous dress

Use this color for accent pieces—blouses, silk shells, and a camisole, for example. You may wish to use this color on your main list as well since it is very powerful for you.

YOUR ACCENT STYLE

A Dramatic may borrow from other style types, but she'll always make them hers. She's the one who will borrow from everyone and keep her accessories flamboyant and wild.

> **Note:** Dramatic contains so many elements of Traditional and Classic that anything here only downplays Ms. Dramatic. These two styles she'll borrow to tone down her look.

Sporty

Accenting with Sporty means looking the part more than being it. A sailor suit is only to wear on the yacht, never to use. Accents relating to her current sport, a nice new ski suit or running shoes, for example. A fancy headband to accent an outfit.

Romantic

Sexy lace and lingerie are borrowed from Romantic here. A lace camisole to wear under a jacket or a long silk dress are also borrowed from Ms. Romantic. However, it is important to keep in mind that a Dramatic is only borrowing Romantic's love of soft feminine details, but it is not her style. Dramatic uses the feminine touches to draw attention to herself and feel sexy in her clothes.

Dramatic

This is the only real accent that a Dramatic has. She is already heavily mortgaged to Classic and Traditional, borrowing their looks and making them showy. Ms. Dramatic has a natural accent.

Trendy

This is the one accent that Ms. Dramatic will consistently try to borrow from, always trying to be ahead of the game, yet she is really more of a upscale Classic.

The problem here is that there is an inherent difference with these two styles. Ms. Dramatic craves attention, while Ms. Trendy could take it or leave it. The idea of throwing something on and not caring appeals to Ms. D., and with this accent it works.

COLOR WITH YOUR OWN PERSONAL STYLE

Dramatic brings her flair for the wild to whatever color she chooses to wear.

A Red Outfit

Pure red is powerful on a Dramatic woman. A red outfit, like her, is a real showstopper. This is the woman who has no fear of criticism and may actually enjoy creating a little scandal. It makes the statement: "I am here to entertain a bit, play a bit, and challenge a bit."

A Dramatic woman may wear this color to a divorce hearing, whether or not she won the settlement, *or* to a gathering at Joan Collins's house.

An Orange Outfit

Many Dramatics have some imbalance with orange. Typically, Dramatics make a show of physical activity, but generally they abhor anything that has to do with physical movement. Appearance and self-care are often a battle when there is an imbalance of orange.

Dramatics express their warmth to masses rather than individuals, so this is not the color she would typically reach for. However, with Dramatics, I often recommend they wear something in the orange family around their close friends and loved ones. It helps radiate a warmth they may feel but be unable to express.

A Yellow Outfit

When Ms. Dramatic is feeling reasonable, she will be in yellow. She'll wear this color to let you know that she will be cooperating today. When she dons yellow, she says: "I'm feeling cooperative, but please be intelligent in your communication."

A Green Outfit

When Ms. Dramatic feels prosperous, she'll reach for something green—to tell the world that the deal has come through and she's off to celebrate!

Her sense of sisterhood is definitely sparked by her feeling of prosperity. A heightened sense of caring for her fellows is one of the strong messages of green when worn by her.

She may turn up at a charity benefit wearing green as well. The key is that she'll often wear green when she is feeling *emotionally* generous.

A Blue Outfit

"Of course I'm telling you the truth, I enjoy being outspoken," says Ms. Dramatic. As loyal as she can be, as much as she desires to communicate—that is her message. Ms. Dramatic chooses blue to indicate confidence, and

she has plenty of it to go around. Others sense it when she wears blue.

She'll show up at a banquet in a beautiful cobalt sequined gown or on her first day of filming, she'll wear her *power* blue suit. (And I mean P-O-W-E-R.)

An Indigo Outfit

Firm in her convictions, direct in her approach, and unchallenged is the message of Ms. Dramatic in indigo.

She is feeling centered from a very high place when she wears indigo, and others will not challenge her, for they too sense that something they cannot see is at work. The magic of indigo on Ms. D is that it mixes the purity of intuition with her direct approach.

A Purple Outfit

Ms. Dramatic's love of lavishness finds her at ease with the extravagant purple. Since purple still has a noble quality, she is naturally drawn to it. The elements that you would use to describe a Dramatic woman are also used to describe purple—regal, respected, and distinguished. Liz Taylor's first perfume, Passion, was marketed in purple packaging—a perfect match!

Ms. Dramatic strengthens her own aura of nobility when she dons purple. Since she loves being revered, wearing purple will draw those to her that admire her. She will definitely show up at a book signing in purple—her autobiography, of course.

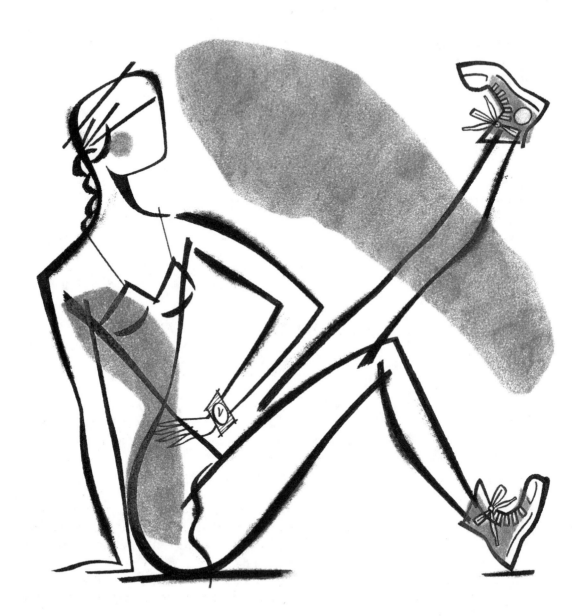

Chapter Nine

TRENDY

The first thing you must understand about a Trendy woman is that she *is* the "trend." This woman sets trends, she doesn't follow them. She'll order pizza in rather than go to that new chic pizza place in town, which she finds boring. She makes a place fashionable by going there.

She's the one who challenges conventional thinking by her actions. Trendy would never scream victim; she isn't afraid to speak up and voice her opinions.

While Ms. Trendy is flexible, she is not at ease working in corporate America. This woman doesn't fit into anyone's mold and has her own ideas about life. Other people's "opinions" have little or no effect on her actions or life choices.

Trendy surprises others by her choices. She may be married one minute, then dating a man twenty years younger the next. Then she'll be pregnant and decide to marry someone other than the baby's father.

One thing is certain: she does not lack morals. She has a strong sense of justice and tries to live her life by that ideal. She is fair and honest and sometimes intimidates others with her frankness! But it doesn't bother her, so why bother changing it?

She makes her decisions based on what she feels is right. This woman lives to be free, and in so doing often inspires others to do the same. She is a leader and is not afraid of doing what feels right to her. She will let her feelings be known (or not known) as it suits her, either way is okay with her.

Trendy is never afraid to be part of something that she believes in. She normally doesn't pay much attention to others—not because she's uncaring, but because she's too involved in whatever is currently happening.

This woman would rather spend a Saturday afternoon visiting an elderly relative than having tea with a diplomat. She has a very clear sense of herself and others' judgments don't effect her. You won't find her preaching on a corner, it's not her style; she lives her beliefs. She's bold, innovative, and not afraid to experiment. That's Trendy!

Clothing? Whatever suits her. Her clothes work for her; she dresses for herself, not to impress others.

Donna Karan typifies Trendy. She designs styles that are simple and individual.

RECOGNIZING A TRENDY

Ms. Trendy completes the style wheel, and rightly so, for she is a conglomeration of all that has come before her, and at the same time, none of those things.

If she's unconventional, then she's Trendy!

She is so changeable that it truly is hard to peg her. Although it is easy to spot what's not her.

She is not any one style long enough to make it hers.

Demi Moore in *The Butcher's Wife* is a perfect example of a mismatched Trendy. She played a romantic style type and was playing against her natural trendy style. While a romantic actress may have fit the role more, the mismatch actually worked in the context of this film because her character really was out of place. The whole idea of a stranger in a strange land worked here. In her roles in both *Ghost* and *Indecent Proposal*, she played Trendys and matched her roles perfectly.

Cher in the movie *Mask* was matched to her role. The character she portrayed lived her life on her own terms and broke rules to do what she felt was right. A powerful, stirring movie was heightened by the match of a Trendy woman playing a trendy role. Perfect.

Bette Midler in her stirring performance in *The Rose* captured our attention instantly. She too has always commanded a career on her own terms, always doing what she feels to be important.

And who else but Madonna could have pulled off a movie like *Truth or Dare?* Doing the unexpected, showing the world who she is in a daring, touching way. The level of intimacy she expects and gives is intimidating to some. This is indicative of a Trendy woman.

Trendy's are deeply involved in life. They typically live so fully that they sometimes shock the rest of the world by their choices. The vivid image of a pregnant Demi Moore on the cover of Vanity Fair comes to mind.

The memorable film roles these Trendy women have portrayed are trendy because they've reached into the depths of their souls and shown us what's inside. There are many Trendys who may never create award-winning film roles or win elections, but you will find them where you least expect to.

What are the elements that make an outfit trendy?

Now that you recognize a Trendy, you can understand my dilemma in showing you what would be a Trendy. However, there are a few tricks that many Trendy's pull, and I'll try and reveal them to you. First, the innate ability to mix her laid-back nature with a dramatic look is one aspect of what makes her Trendy.

Keep in mind that there is always an edge to Trendy that would even be too wild for her Dramatic sister. Unlike Dramatic, who wants to be admired, Trendy loves to raise questions, prompt discussions, and fire up controversy. She enjoys being noticed, but what she chooses to wear is not based upon your opinion, only hers.

What is the difference between Dramatic and Trendy? Dramatic has a "notice me, I look fabulous" quality to any outfit she wears. Trendy is always eclectic. The attitude is carefree. The shorts are too short to be functional and the skirts are too long to be in proportion. In short, Trendy is a rule breaker or boundary pusher. She likes to experiment and see how far she can get.

Things that mismatch are Trendy. Short boots and bulky socks with a dress are definite mismatches and elements that create Trendy. She is too sexy to be a Sporty, and too carefree to be a Dramatic. How can you spot a Trendy? Look for the mix of Dramatic and Sporty.

Anything she wears will take on its own flair.

A TRENDY STORY

I met Chloe a few years ago after she attended one of my fashion seminars. She was wearing a beige linen baggy pant cinched at the waist with a large brown belt. Her pants were capri length, and she was wearing a traditional white button-down oxford blouse.

She struck up a conversation with me telling me how lucky I was to be independent and "doing my own thing." She admired my sky blue suit, telling me that the company she worked with was so traditional that "the only blue anyone wears is navy."

She was an architect working in a very traditional firm and said she had reached the point where she "hated" her job.

In speaking to her, it became clear to me that the only way she was going to be happy was to either find a company that was more trendy (since she was a trendy) or start her own business.

Would I, she asked, "sort out my hodge-podge wardrobe and make me look like I belong somewhere." The quiz revealed that she *was* a true Trendy. Her wardrobe was supposed to be hodgepodge.

CLOSET OR COLLAGE?

Chloe brought her collage to our first meeting. I hadn't recalled telling her to do one yet. But she explained that I'd told her about it when we first met and she figured she'd just get a jump on the work.

Her collage was filled with buildings that created her own unique skyline. Interspersed with the skyscrapers were pictures of museums and buildings that fascinated her. A few homes were also in the picture. Why?

She loved architecture.

In her statement she mentioned her traditional mother, and I surmised that this was a key factor in her gravitating toward a more conservative work environment.

From both her collage and statement it was clear that she loved her work, but the environment didn't suit her. She was ready to quit her job. I suggested she wait. At least until we worked on her closet.

COLORS IN HER CLOSET

Once I saw the contents of her closet, I nixed the idea of having her redo her collage.

This woman knew her style. She knew who she was, she just hadn't found the right environment yet.

Her feelings about the seasonal color theory were typically trendy. She didn't like to follow a particular formula when it came to her colors, only what worked for her.

However, pumpkin, icy yellow, and black were the dominant colors in her wardrobe. When I pressed her to categorize her three personal colors, she came up with the following:

1. Icy yellow was the color she felt best wearing (how she sees herself),
2. Pumpkin was the color she received the most compliments on, (how the world sees her), and
3. Black was the color she felt powerful wearing.

Knowing she was an autumn helped me because I needed to assist her in adding color into her wardrobe.

Why an autumn? In general, the color you receive the most compliments on will be on your seasonal chart.

In Chloe's case, pumpkin fell into the autumn chart and it made sense to me. For Chloe was working in an environment that wasn't her and wore colors that weren't her. The biggest clue came when I began to study her personal colors.

Icy yellow was another indication that she was cutting herself off from the work she loved. She was not feeling very cooperative and was having a hard time with the teamwork that her job entailed. This color was a strong indication that she was feeling displaced.

Pumpkin actually gave me the strongest indication of who she was. Chloe was a powerful woman who could easily inspire others. She was much better in small groups and was probably held in high regard by her colleagues.

And, finally black is all about the need to be taken seriously.

Like a true Trendy, I suspected that these colors would change as she made changes in her life. Except for the color she received the most compliments on. This color tends not to change for any of us, since it is the most natural one we wear.

I now understood why she wore only black to work. The first and most obvious reason was she could get away with wearing much more trendy styles in black than she could wearing a color.

Surrounded by a family of scientists, her creative, trendy style made Chloe the oddball.

So it was not a huge surprise to find that her home was black and modern and she drove a black car.

THE SHOPPING LIST

Chloe had some work to do, and I assured her that we would take it slow so she'd feel comfortable. Being a Trendy, her response was, "No way! Let's change it now. Why wait?" I suggested we start where she had wanted to: with the hodgepodge collection in her closet.

Once inside the thrift store that she called a closet (or as my best friend says, a "Classic's nightmare"), I had to go back to my original thought about her. Chloe did not need a new wardrobe; she needed an environment where she could fully be herself. After she realized how appropriate her clothes were for her, her work environment was exactly what she changed. Six months after we met, Chloe opened up her own firm and today is very successful in her business.

Yes, I know, a happy ending. But how did we handle her thrift store wardrobe?

THE RESULTS

We went on a shopping spree right in her closet. Things that no longer suited her were dispensed with. We found a few things that she no longer wore and we resurrected them.

Instead of a shopping list, we created a list from what was already there.

What exactly was in her closet? Tons of black. Almost two-thirds of her wardrobe was made up of black outfits, and most of her accessories were silver or black-and-white geometrics.

1. Two pairs of trousers, one in black with suspenders and the other in taupe with a paperbag waist

2. Workshirts in yellow and pumpkin to wear with the pants

3. Funky suspenders in patterns that worked in with her trousers

4. Two linen jackets that also worked in here

5. A pair of eyeglasses in pumpkin. I encouraged her to get another pair in olive. She did. This was before I discovered that she

didn't really need glasses, she just liked to wear them as an accessory. Trendy.

Interestingly she had never worn any of the above items together.

6. She owned a stretch-lace black dress that fit her fabulously. It fell to her ankles, and over it she layered a white blouse with more bangles than I could count. And, some black lace-up boots, very romantic!

7. Quite a few knit outfits in black. Long slinky dresses that were sporty knits; she could wear her sweaters over these or tie them with a few of her belts. This woman owned the most incredible original belt designs I'd ever seen.

With all of these things she wore her lace-up boots. In the summer she could wear a pair of sneakers. That was her work wardrobe.

Her casual wardrobe was thrift-store chic. We also added a few pieces, and she naturally was drawn to warm autumn tones.

1. A new floral dress in a design with warm tones
2. A few summer hats
3. She agreed to add one DKNY item every month to her wardrobe as a basic.
4. A pair of wild metallic shoes. They were platforms, and I can tell you that I'd never wear them, but on her—Wow! She found these antiques in a thrift store.
5. A mustard yellow suit. She already owned a black cape that made this suit scream trendy! And it looked sensational on her.
6. A kooky space suit with zippers and gadgets on it. It was funky and wild, and it was in a rust color. She found it at a French boutique.

My work with Chloe helped her gain insight into the fact that she already was a style. She hadn't needed to conform to someone else's idea of what was "fashionable." What Chloe needed was to impress upon her business clients that she was innovative and confident when it came to designing structures. In taking inventory of her wardrobe, she realized that her clothing did just that. It wasn't hard for me to see that in her own business she would thrive because anyone would definitely trust this gutsy lady when it came to designing an "original" home for them.

TRENDYS IN THE WORK FORCE

If you're seeking a conformist or a "yes" person, *don't hire this woman! Innovative, provocative, argumentative, peaceful* are words that all describe Ms. T!

To stay employed, she must feel free to express herself in her work environment—or she will anyway.

Ms. Trendy has such a hard time following others' rules that she rarely is "employed" for long. If she stays somewhere, it is because the boss has given up on trying to change her, and she's such a valuable addition to the company they put up with her.

Many Trendys have had legions of jobs, others simply own their own companies to avoid the boss issue altogether.

Many clothing designers are Trendys themselves for they are free spirits who live life on terms that defy normal work conditions.

Dedicated and impassioned, Trendy will risk her career over "rights," hers or another persons. She knows that doing unto others is the only way to work and live.

INTO YOUR CLOSET FOR SPECIAL OCCASIONS

1. White Tie—

Some of the most outlandish ball gowns I've ever seen have been worn by Trendy women. This really is a hard call to make without knowing you.

Trendy wardrobes vary so greatly, my only suggestion is that if you are concerned about what you are wearing, ask. Most Trendys don't really care for an outside opinion, so they wear whatever they wish and civilians gawk.

2. Black Tie—

I've seen a Trendy wear short shorts in black with lace stockings, black army boots, and a tuxedo jacket with cummerbund, the works, on top.

I thought she looked great, although some didn't feel that she was wearing appropriate attire and snickered. In truth, this is meant to be formal, and since you wear formal for casual and vice versa, there may be something already in your closet that is more than appropriate for black tie.

The fact remains that Trendy is still not a conformist and would rather wear black tie to a museum than to an event that requires it. So for you a quick trip to a thrift store or an outrageous boutique might uncover something that suits you.

3. Black Tie Optional—

Anything goes for you here. You probably can already put together something that would shock, and far surpass what anyone else has on.

4. Cocktail Reception—

Only you can really decide what your comfort level is at one of these events. I've seen Trendys in everything from torn jeans to a formal gown. Your attire must match your current mood.

Remember, Trendys dress the unexpected.

Also, whether you choose any of your personal colors is up to you. This will depend upon the group you'll be mingling with. It's not always appropriate to wear your personal colors. Sometimes, borrowing from another style type is a fabulous option for you.

A TRAVELING TRENDY

For you, travel packing can be a menace. Try to find six to eight pieces that work together so you aren't bringing everything you own with you.

Keep in mind that every Trendy has a different signature piece. For Chloe it was her lace-up boots. They worked into almost everything in her wardrobe. If you build your travel ensemble around your signature piece, you can learn to travel light.

The hardest part about providing a packing list for a Trendy woman is that two different Trendys could have completely different lists. My friend Victoria is a true Trendy. When I asked her to make up a list for me, she phoned me and told me that there were only a few things. Typical Trendy! What follows are the "few things" Victoria travels with. Since she is an actress, she has no need for business suits.

Victoria's list for a seven-day business trip:

a) Straw hat
b) Sunglasses
c) Two patterned scarves to wear Marilyn Monroe–style on her head
d) Four white tank tops
e) Two dress shorts
f) One hiking short
g) One outdoor short
h) Four skirts: two long, two short
i) Two dresses: one with sleeves, one without sleeves
j) Two pants: one patterned, one white

k) One sweater
l) One jacket (rainproof)
m) One pair flat sandals
n) Two pairs low-heeled shoes. Slingbacks. If there are cobblestones there, no heels.
o) Two boots: one dress boot, one pair hiking boots
p) Running shoes
q) A watch, a necklace, a few rings. Not much jewelry.
r) Literature, photos, and my dogs

Going to the beach? Add a bathing suit

TOWN OR COUNTRY?

A Trendy woman can be confirmed city folk, career woman, the whole thing, then a week later become a married country farmer.

Always up to the unexpected, no matter where she lives. By the way, you can bet her neighbors know who she is. She's the neighbor they're all talking about.

An important fashion note: no matter what, Ms. Trendy is fiercely protective of her own rights (as well as others'), and being a nonconformist, there's really no telling what would be right for her.

The only key to her style is that she's between Dramatic and Sporty on the wheel, needing both attention and activity.

TRENDY WARDROBE BASICS

1. Take a solid inventory of your wardrobe. Do clean out your closet. There is a good possibility that most of what you own is already appropriate for you.
2. Work with your personal colors only if it suits you.
3. A new hat is always a good plan for you.
4. Something very forward—remember, you lead trends. Cher wore sheer before sheer was the rage. Madonna wore bra tops and she started a trend! You often know what is coming in next year and wear it early, while the rest of us just stare. Either that or you create and *set* the trends. Remember that many designers are Trendys.
5. A pair of pants in an unexpected fabric or color.
6. A dress. Something unexpected. Since travel is important to you, an item that travels well.
7. Jeans. Something with patches, crochet, suede, or cutouts.
8. You may need to add a new shoe silhouette or something dated like a pair of 1940s-style pumps. Because shoes are important to you. (A pair of funky wild sneakers to wear with jeans may work.)
9. A pair of very trendy sunglasses.
10. A new addition to your (already outrageous) jewelry collection. A pin that is fabulous or a great watch. Whatever it is, it'll be unique and eye-catching.

YOUR ACCENT STYLE

A Trendy will use whatever suits her, often mixing styles to come up with something so unique that it matches her. However, she may choose a style to accent with. Don't forget to read the style chapter about your accent.

Sporty

Many of the sporty elements of this style type are already in your wardrobe. Funky keys on a silver chain, shoes that are sporty, and comfortable clothes that are primarily weekend wear will line your closet.

Your life-style will tend to be that of an artist or designer if your accent is here. For your clothing will be very casual. Accessorizing will be functional, a whistle on a chain, a bag with a small umbrella compartment built in.

Romantic

Floppy hats and romantic dresses may find their way easily into your closet. You will tend to use interesting mixes of lace and soft fabrics. Accessories will be soft feminine pieces. Pearls will work easily for you, or soft crushed-velvet bags.

Traditional

Jessica Lange falls into this category. While this woman does her own thing, she also values and respects traditional family values. Brave, solid, and dependable, a Trendy whose accents are traditional will always be thrust into the limelight for her unconventional life-style, while on a very deep level she herself is very conventional. Her strong need to break free every now and then is evidenced in the way she does what suits her, but never, ever at the expense of her family or someone else.

Accessorizing will be simple: an antique pin, a hat with flowers, something that adds a sense of a long-ago time to the newness of Trendy.

Classic

If you're running a business, you may wind up with quite a few Anne Klein jewelry pieces in your wardrobe. To accent with Classic is to be crisp, bold, and clean in your choices.

Your accessories will be fashionable, high-priced items that you will tire of long before they go out of style.

Dramatic

What was once "old" becomes new here. The chiffon scarf with starlet glasses is only one example of the unexpected results from this combination.

Remember that Trendy can show up wearing anything, surprising even her own family. Now add any *dramatic* element to this mix. Accessories will be polished and flashy. And as always, unexpected.

Trendy

Bette Midler is a pure Trendy. This personality takes life on her own terms. She will rise or fall according to her own whims of the moment. She changes based upon what her present needs are and isn't afraid of taking a 180-degree turn on any opinion she currently has.

Accessories will run the gamut from pearls to studs and leather. She can show up wearing anything at anytime.

COLOR WITH YOUR OWN PERSONAL STYLE

Trendy brings her flair for the unexpected to any color she chooses to wear.

A Red Outfit

This look is fun and extremely strong. It screams individualism more than any other color. This color tells the world that you will be a star despite bad press.

A Trendy woman would wear red to an opening night party *or* to dinner with her parents when she tells them that she is moving to Cuba and taking up the cause.

An Orange Outfit

"I am here. And I am involved!" says Ms. Trendy as she enters the room wearing orange. Her warmth and ability to "dig in" are apparent in orange.

She will appear wearing orange at a protest where there are others who share her beliefs. (Incidentally, she is very capable of *starting* and organizing a protest as well.) In orange, her spirit and energy motivate others.

A Yellow Outfit

Stand up and scream, "This is what I think!" and you'll get the fun witty feeling of Trendy in yellow.

Since this is the color of intellect, a Trendy will wear this without hesitation, for her thinking is immediate. She doesn't need to belabor things.

Her rationale, whether or not you agree with her, is hers and hers alone. She is the style innovator and yellow is about innovative thinking. Expect the unexpected from Ms. Outspoken.

A Green Outfit

Green + Ms. Trendy = a heightening of her own growth or self-awareness. A Trendy woman strongly believes in universal love and sisterhood. While she may do things that seem to be self-fulfilling, there is always a greater good in the back of her mind.

When Ms. Trendy puts green on, it is about her own personal growth. Like the leaves on a tree, a Trendy woman growing will reach for this color. This is how she lets others know that she is learning something in the emotional area.

A Trendy will often choose green when she mourns or grieves, because it is the color close to her heart.

A Blue Outfit

If Ms. Trendy shows up wearing blue, you can bet it is to express herself. Since she communicates in her own style, you can count on the fact that the way she wears blue is just as individual.

She may wear a sky blue outfit with ruffles or lace to a black tie dinner (and look stunning), or a *real* navy blue "sailor" suit to go on a yacht.

Since her style is her own, that's just how she'll wear the communication color: her very own way.

An Indigo Outfit

An unwavering faith is indicated when Ms. Trendy steps out in indigo. She has aligned herself with a truth (of her own) and is steadfast in her beliefs.

Since indigo signifies our intuition, when Ms. Trendy wears indigo, she is very powerful indeed, for she thrives on her intuition. Her intuition is the most valuable resource for a Trendy woman and is closely aligned with her beliefs, allowing her to act in a way that she perceives as correct.

A Purple Outfit

Ms. Trendy finds the spirituality she craves in purple—although count on her to wear this color in unexpected ways to unusual places.

This could be the color she wears to learn to milk a cow or to go to church, for Ms. Trendy perceives life as a spiritual experience. *Spiritual* is definitely the key word to associate with Ms. Trendy in purple.

Purple could make her appear distant or aloof to others when she wears it, even though that may not be her intent. No matter what, she is always respected when she wears purple.

Chapter Ten

MOTHERS AND DAUGHTERS

If you grew up with a mother who was a different style type, there were probably more than a few confusing moments.

Quite frequently, mothers define the accent type most women have, but this is not an absolute. There are times when another person can influence our accent style.

I find it helpful to understand the dynamics between mother and daughter style types to better comprehend your own style and evolution.

A SPORTY MOTHER

When Mom's a Sporty, whether on the slopes for skiing, on the green for golf, or sampling the newest restaurant in town, she's probably the first in line for a new adventure. Never frail or helpless, she wouldn't let you be lazy either; she's ever the coach, always encouraging. Health and activity are just another fact of life for her.

If she does lose her temper, it's generally because she's frustrated. When she finds something she doesn't understand, it is in her nature to try to grasp it. If she can't, she gets upset.

When challenged with a style type differing from her own, she may be lost.

THE DAUGHTERS

Sporty

This child is so much like her mother, she may struggle with her own sense of femininity from time to time. They could wind up as doubles partners at tennis; if not that, definitely partners in some kind of sport.

Sharing a similar life-style, they will share similar wardrobe problems and pluses as well. They will have a functional wardrobe, but not necessarily one that works for everything. Seeking out a Classic relative for wardrobe advice can be helpful, but you must, remember to keep your focal point Sporty.

Romantic

Sporty will connect with Romantic. These two will enjoy most pursuits that have to do with land or sea.

While it would seem at first that their styles are as different as night and day, that is not true. Sporty and Romantic both belong to the mutual admiration society, for Sporty will admire Romantic's feminine style and Romantic will appreciate Sporty's spunk!

Keep in mind that while a Romantic may find a dress for the Renaissance Fair a necessity, Sporty may find some of her romantic notions fanciful.

Sporty will appreciate her daughter's delicate taste and may share some elements of her daughter's wardrobe with her.

Traditional

Here comes a role reversal! While a Traditional may never hike to the top of Mount Everest with her mother, she can appreciate the benefits of a good walk.

Sporty may wish her Traditional daughter were more "competitive," but Traditional simply is not as active as her mother is and may never be; this could be a source of frustration for the two of them. Traditional's intellectual pursuits and Sporty's active life could create a wonderful relationship between them since they'd have much to share.

Classic

A Classic will be involved in activities because of her mother's influence. A Classic daughter will desire to look good participating in Sporty's skiing or horseback riding, almost to the point of feeling overdone to her mother.

This is a good growth match. They each admire the other's style, but Classic will need to buy expensive clothes and Sporty won't understand that. Classic's promise to take care of her things and wear them for a long time may fall on deaf ears, since Sporty wears clothes until they rip apart.

Expensive, high-quality clothes for everyday wear are perfect for a Classic. Sporty may need to allow her daughter the luxury of buying expensive clothes that don't make sense to her, but to her daughter are important. Sporty can learn from Classic about proper business wear, and Classic can learn to play from her mom.

Dramatic

Sporty will be at a loss here. She won't understand why a walk in the country won't make her little Dramatic feel better.

Dramatic may crave clothes that simply don't appear functional to her mother: *"Where do you plan to wear that?"* may be the question in a common refrain.

Okay, so wearing a red dress with matching sandals to school could be a mite eccentric. Dramatic's first thought is not to be a participant, it's to be the show. What is really key here is that for a Sporty mom, it's impossible for her to really comprehend owning clothes that are anything other than useful.

Sporty may feel completely ill-equipped to help a Dramatic daughter with clothing, but she will definitely come to appreciate her when she has a formal occasion to go to. This child will know exactly what to suggest!

Trendy

Sporty may not understand Trendy's gift of making herself over constantly. Although she will appreciate Trendy's ability to master whatever she has her heart into. They share an uncanny ability to adapt to any situation emotionally, as well as the ability to work extremely hard at whatever they undertake.

A ROMANTIC MOTHER

Lucky is the child who has a Romantic mother! For her focus in life is always love first. Romantic is often so successful at whatever career she chooses, she balances home and career well. A Romantic mother will put a successful career on hold if she feels that her children need her. She is in touch with her children and makes every attempt to stay close.

THE DAUGHTERS

Sporty

Oops! This child will fight those frilly dresses every inch of the way! Put her in one, and she'll come back with it torn, or filthy, or both. She's the child who gets scrapes and bruises constantly.

Sporty loves to wear clothes that set her free to participate in life the way she chooses. Romantic can understand the need to feel good in clothing. If Romantic allows Sporty to wear the functional clothes she chooses, she may surprise her mother by choosing to one day show up for tea and crumpets. (Don't worry, she'll wear a dress).

Romantic

Heaven. Very little can separate this duo. They both understand the importance of their relationship and will let nothing come between them. This child will gain so very much from her mother, who in turn will have a closeness that she's never before had. This relationship is the one a Romantic woman has been searching for.

Traditional

This child will be Romantic's pride and joy. She is well behaved and will dress slightly more conservatively than her Romantic mom, but nonetheless, Romantic will appreciate her calming manner.

However, since Traditional relies heavily on her family, she may never cut the home ties fully and set out into the world like the other style types. She may choose or opt for a more traditional career that has a family atmosphere.

Traditional is also proper and respectful, qualities that a Romantic can nurture and appreciate.

Classic

It may be hard for Romantic to understand her Classic daughter. For Classic's focus is not love first. Classic's work will come first and missed meals at home may leave her mother feeling wounded. Romantic Mom may feel family must come first, and will have to try to understand that she did nothing wrong in raising a child so different from her. While Classic loves her family, it may not be in the sacrificing way Romantic feels that it should be.

On the very positive side, Romantic is quite the perfect mother for a Classic child, who will learn from her mother how to love and be there for others. With a solid base of love behind her, Classic has a good foundation to carry out into the world.

While they may approach life from opposite extremes, they tend to value the same things.

Dramatic

Romantic will encourage self-expression in her daughter, although she may put her foot down where propriety is concerned.

Dramatic's flamboyant manner could ruffle Romantic's feathers from time to time. Romantic will need to accept Dramatic's style or she may find herself at odds with her daughter.

Letting Dramatic find creative outlets that appeal to her will strengthen their relationship and help Dramatic to focus all her wild energy.

Trendy

There may be times when Romantic is astounded by her daughter's sense of style. It's important to realize that while Trendy will appreciate love and attention, Romantic can't expect the same from her. At least not in the same way. Doting is simply not her.

Her clothes will change with her moods, and just when you think you know her—Whamo!—she's made a total transformation right before your eyes.

If a Trendy child wants to paint the walls of her room black, it may appall Romantic, but she had best avoid telling Trendy that she'll tire of it in two months. She will, and already she knows it. (This isn't a threat to Trendy, who isn't afraid of making herself over at the drop of a hat.) Don't think her putting delicate floral wallpaper over those black walls means she's changed. Trendy will be onto something else before Romantic has even grown accustomed to the last thing.

The marvelous thing about a Trendy child is that she won't worry about being "right." She knows that she'll outgrow a phase, but she realizes that this is no reason to skip it.

These two can really be close, since they can enjoy a strong sense of humor.

A TRADITIONAL MOTHER

Since tradition and family go hand in hand for a Traditional mom, she is the best suited of all the style types to be a parent. She is accepting and supportive and perhaps more trusting than she should be.

However, instilling her beliefs in her own children, however noble they may be, has its downside, too. Many children of Traditional moms wind up feeling immense guilt over being anything other than what their mom wants them to be.

THE DAUGHTERS

Sporty

Perhaps one of the greatest style clashes of all, these two could be surprisingly close, regardless.

While Traditional will tend to put Sporty in dresses when she's young and try to teach her to be a "lady," this child will be busy trying to figure out how she can escape and go play. Any attempts at taming Sporty could cause a wedge between them. However, her mom's humility and family values will be respected by Sporty. Traditional and Sporty share much in the way of beliefs and values, and can be quite close in that respect.

There is another benefit to a Sporty daughter: she's low maintenance! Just buy her a pair of jeans and let her become whoever she is meant to be. Traditional can outfit her daughter in Guess or Esprit and off she'll go.

Sporty may wind up occasionally getting into a beautiful traditional dress—with her hiking boots, of course.

Romantic

Fairy tales and love are Romantic's whimsy. Traditional believes that love is sacrifice and compromise. Therein lies the natural conflict between these two types.

While Traditional's values will be appreciated by Romantic, but she doesn't believe in giving up love for anything.

Good feelings are everything to this child. She will actively pursue love and passionate friendships. If love is gone, then so is the Romantic. She's the one who disappears when family arguments erupt.

There is much to learn from a Romantic daughter. How to enjoy life, for one. She naturally avoids the "harsh realities of life" that Traditional faces. Romantic children *should* be allowed to pursue their dreams, for many become quite successful in the arts—where dreams are made into reality.

Traditional

A Traditional child may not try to stretch herself and discover much outside her family if she shares a style type with her mom. After all, home is cozy and safe, why go elsewhere?

Rules and regulations are very natural to her, and she is the joy of her family.

Traditionals with Traditional moms tend to marry young, choosing to follow in their mother's footsteps. Traditional mothers are such wonderful role models that their daughters wants what their mother has. Their styles are so identical that they have fun shopping together, cooking together, and sharing many other things including interests such as literature and art.

Classic

A Classic child will be so absorbed in whatever she is doing, she may forget to set the table when told. She'll forget because family chores just don't carry the weight to her that they do to her mom. A Classic will be the first to hire someone to handle domestic duties for her, because she gets too caught up in work and other interests to pay attention to it.

Unfortunately, a Traditional places a great deal of emphasis on the amount other members of her family contribute to the whole, and this child may come up short by her standards. Classic simply doesn't measure love the same way. There will be bridges to cross here, but Traditional's love and understanding will help close the gap.

In addition, Classic may spend large sums of money on her clothing, which may seem unnecessary to her Traditional mother. Although Traditional will admire her daughter's polish and ability to always be "in" fashion. When Classic assures her mother that she will wear some of those items for years, she isn't lying, she really will.

Dramatic

Oh boy! Traditional mothers often have trouble with a free life-style. The good side is that Traditional will get out more with a Dramatic daughter!

From the moment she learns to talk, Dramatic will want to help her mom coordinate a wardrobe. Attire is not at the top of Traditional's priority list, and she may wonder why it is for her daughter. To Dramatic, being noticed is very important.

Dramatic will bring out the daring side of her mother, and these two could have lots of fun together. Dramatic will put up with her mother's comments about wild clothing, because underneath all that is a woman who

fiercely loves her mother. The feelings are mutual.

Trendy

Traditional's eyes will stay wide open where her little Trendy is concerned! This child will change like the weather in the tropics, and in attempting to keep up with her, Traditional could drive herself mad!

Traditional may not understand how anything remotely coordinated will come out of her daughter's closet. It won't take much to discover that Traditional and her daughter are as different as two people can be.

Trendy will always understand her mother, and quite often her wardrobe will contain major pieces that are Traditional. As opposites on the wheel, they only appear diametrically opposed. In actuality, Trendy will gain much in the way of values and loyalty from her Traditional mother. The conservative Traditional, on the other hand, will learn to let go a little more. These two can be very close, enjoying each other and shopping.

A CLASSIC MOTHER

Because Ms. Classic has run the show for so long, it's hard for her to let go and focus on her family. Since she is wrapped around her career, she may not understand a child who differs from her. Classic has a hard time accepting that a style other than her own *is* a style.

This is a woman whom people respect as an individual in her own right. She may even be more successful than her mate. She is a clotheshorse and knows how to shop.

THE DAUGHTERS

Sporty

Now here's a combo that amuses Ms. Classic! When her daughter shows up in ripped jeans, Classic may want to smooth out what she sees as a diamond in the rough. Sporty will admire her mother's style and adopt a few touches for her own. It's very common for a Sporty with a Classic mom to adopt her mother's accent style quite strongly.

Sporty will come out with some odd combinations that somehow look great on her, many of which her mother knows shouldn't work but appreciates. This child will definitely challenge her mother's own personal sense of style. They will come to appreciate their opposite qualities of work and play, each learning from the other.

Romantic

This child could confuse a Classic mother. The way she feels in her clothing is far more important to a Romantic than a polished look. It's not uncommon for Ms. Classic to feel badly for her Romantic daughter, whom she feels has no clothes.

Her little Romantic, who's only concern is love, will admire her mom and appreciate everything she does. A Classic mom will have to work at understanding that her daughter is different from her, and accept that.

Romantic and Classic can become very close, for Romantic will teach her mother how important love is.

Traditional

She may not share her mother's appreciation of clothing, for her values are different than Ms. Classic's. A Traditional child will spend her time with friends or in quiet activities. She may enjoy cooking and reading so much that to a Classic mother, it can appear to be excessive.

The Traditional child accepts her mother's being slightly more flamboyant than she and admires her mother's style. Ms. Classic will come to love her daughters quiet loyalty. A Traditional child has much to teach Classic about loyalty and parenting, for she is much more patient than her mother.

Classic

For a Classic, there is nothing better than someone who shares her taste! Except someone who shares her taste.

The only real problem for these two can arise if they are the same size. Then each of them will have to protect their possessions. Otherwise they can expect to be shopping pals!

Dramatic

A Dramatic's ability to outshine her mother from a very early age is something that will unnerve her Classic mother. This child will pick outfits that come as a constant surprise; while some choices will seem questionable, she can and does pull them off.

Her mother will come to understand that a Dramatic is very intuitive about what works and should be given room to wear what matches her personality. They can share a wonderful sense of humor, and Dramatic will learn a powerful work ethic from her mother.

Trendy

Like Dramatic, Trendy will astound her Classic mother with the current color of her hair or the number of earrings she wears. Then one day, she'll stun her mother by wearing a completely classic outfit.

If a child is a chameleon, she's probably a Trendy. Her ability to change herself and reinvent her style is just her gift, not something that needs to be worked out. She's more of a free spirit than Ms. Classic, who may not understand all the changing. Ms. Classic will appreciate, however, her daughter's outspokenness and even encourage it.

Since Classic's focus is work, her daughter will have a Classic work ethic, which can be amazingly powerful for a Trendy. These two will be good friends.

A DRAMATIC MOTHER

A Dramatic mother is the most noticed mom on the block. She is fun, adventurous, and always finds offbeat and unusual activities to share with her children. Her campfire stories are always the best and most fun. She can become very involved with her kids, sometimes inadvertently overshadowing them. In her quest for closeness, she may smother.

She may overlook her daughter's need to be herself, as well as her need for privacy. It may not occur to Dramatic that her children may not be the same as she is.

Of all the style types, Ms. Dramatic will often learn the most *from* her children. Hers is not a style lesson, but a life lesson.

THE DAUGHTERS

Sporty

A Sporty daughter will rarely wear what Mom approves of. In fact, cooperation may be difficult since a Dramatic has a hard time with anyone who doesn't want to do things the way she wants them done. And Sporty is a rebel. Not intentionally, mind you, she just seeks comfort and doesn't understand what all the pomp and circumstance are all about.

A Sporty child will rebel at any attempt to put her in clothing that makes her feel the least bit restricted. Bows fly out of her hair, and Sunday shoes get shed in favor of bare feet or, to any Dramatic's horror, her ruffled socks. Many outfits do wind up ruined by a Sporty child.

Travel is one area where these two will be on equal footing. Sporty can throw on her most comfortable clothing, and with Dramatic in hers, they can stalk adventure around the globe. Dramatic will give her Sporty child a worldliness that she may not get anywhere else. This can be a fun relationship.

From a Dramatic mother, a Sporty child can learn how to add flair to any outfit, as well as how *not* to compromise her position on anything she does.

Romantic

The good thing about this combination is that there will be no mistaking these two styles. What is important here is that Dramatic allow her Romantic daughter to choose what she wants to wear as early as possible. Dramatic may not understand her daughter's choices, or why she needs so much quiet time. But Romantic's daydreams are a part of her makeup. Most Romantics become highly successful in their lives and their melodramas about boys are only part of their journey.

Romantic will admire her mother and allow her to be the center of attention without much friction, and Dramatic appreciates her daughter's sense of romance. Romantic will teach her mother that gentleness is a wonderful quality.

Traditional

Now here's an odd couple! Traditional's basic style will stupefy the Dramatic mom. Dramatic mothers are surprisingly sensitive, but need to be careful not to push a Traditional too hard into the limelight. A Traditional tends to gain attention through academic achievement.

Traditional loves her mother and in many ways will idolize her. Dramatic will accept her daughter and appreciate her loyalty and friendship.

Classic

Dramatic tends to move very quickly through looks and will be quite ahead of others, including her own daughter. While a Classic does share a love of timeless elegance with her mother, she does not share her mother's desire to be the centerpiece.

Dramatic must be conscious of the fact that while her daughter and she are quite close in their style, they still have varying tastes.

These two will teach each other that teamwork has its benefits, it's called friendship.

Dramatic

While their style may be the same, this is not necessarily an idyllic combination! They both need to be the center of attention, and a little competition could flare up. The daughter can feel stifled around her more glamorous mother, and it is to her advantage to find her own crowd of admirers. These two need time apart to appreciate their similar tastes.

On the good side, they can also enjoy sharing the spotlight and creating a stir together. Sharing a style, they intuitively know the other's taste, so shopping for or with each other is easy and fun. They are a powerful mother/daughter team and can be extremely close.

Trendy

Trendy's ability to make herself over will amaze even a Dramatic mother! Dramatic is the woman who thought she had the inside track on everything—imagine her surprise here.

Trendy's way of expressing herself and the way she reinvents her style almost magically will stun her mother. Dramatic will also be impressed by her daughter's nonchalance about her appearance. Whether Trendy looks awesome or dreary won't faze her, she is okay with either state.

Dramatic will appreciate Trendy's adaptability to change. Not phased by her mothers love of the limelight, Trendy can have a warm and close relationship with her mother.

A TRENDY MOTHER

This is a woman who wants her daughter to be whatever she wishes to be. A wonderful thing, but her free, loving nature can make it hard for a child to assert her independence.

Since Trendy express herself, she encourages others to do the same. Her free spirited quality may cause her children to be watchful over *her* at times. Her kids often wind up quite together in spite of her zaniness. She is strict where values are concerned and surrounding the issue of right and wrong.

Her ease with anything she does is typical of a Trendy mother. Trendy's personal confidence is contagious.

Sporty

This child actually has a perfect mother in Trendy. Her seeming lack of femininity won't throw her mother off or make her uncomfortable. Trendy will gallantly defend her child's ripped jeans (and her inability to sit quietly with the girls) to her own mother and friends.

This child needs someone to have the faith in her that Trendy can easily supply. Sporty may draw her Trendy mom into a regular exercise routine. Trendy is willing to spend time with her daughter pursuing her own interests.

Romantic

This child is committed to her femininity, although her consistency in her style may bug the freestyle Trendy. All the lace and feminine stuff is fine for a while, but Mom will hope that her daughter will get over this phase.

She won't.

This is her daughter.

Girlish things appeal to her while Trendy could become impatient with what she considers the "damsel in distress" stuff. If Trendy allows herself to, she may learn quite a bit about love from this child who cherishes all things beautiful, soft, and romantic.

This can be a relationship where both derive quite a bit from each other.

Traditional

There may be times when Trendy feels that her daughter is not stretching her wings wide enough. But this child may be stretching as wide as she can.

Trendy is best at appreciating the differences in people, but she may have a child who is almost too well behaved for her tastes. This is a child who will excel at school and in academics. She is nowhere near as direct as her mother. And, as a result, when she holds things in it may bother a Trendy mother. But this is in a Traditional's nature. If Trendy allows her daughter to open up on her own, this can be a deep friendship.

Classic

Being mistaken for sisters from time to time is quite common for these two. It is Classic's maturity, and Trendy's youth that will close the age gap between them. In truth, Trendy will marvel at her child's ability to always dress well. Classic shops easily in department stores and comes away with wonderful purchases, while her Trendy mother doesn't.

This is a child who instinctively knows

her way around a clothing store with a mother who doesn't think about it much. Trendy won't feel the need to understand her daughter, but she will come to accept her.

Dramatic

This is a click then clash relationship. Trendy doesn't have the need to be "on," like her daughter does. While she may feel that the kid is overdressed from time to time, she'll come to understand that this is simply in her daughter's makeup.

Dramatic will learn from her Trendy mother that everyone needs downtime and Trendy will admire her daughter's flair for fashion. This will be a mutual admiration society and Dramatic can grow quite a bit.

Trendy

Trendy will discover now with just how fiercely independent she was as a child! They both will be very compatible, since the constant change and need to reinvent themselves will not seem strange to each other.

Their shopping strategies will be shared. However, as they already know, there may be times when they are closer than others, based upon what faze they each are going through.

Trendys are impulsive people by nature, and any arguments can be doozies. They will both have to work at controlling their tempers, since this is the only character trait that alienates Trendy from others and Mom won't want to heighten it in her daughter.

Chapter Eleven

THE SIX STYLE TYPES FOR MEN

While I originally designed the style system for women, men can and do fall into the style types as well. Although illustrating how to build a wardrobe using the style types for men is a separate book, I would be remiss to not recognize and address this.

While more and more men are dressing themselves, the primary shopper for a man may be his wife, mother, girlfriend, etc. This section is designed for you, not him.

The six style types are all the same except that **Bohemian** replaces **Romantic.**

Now, the styles for men are: **Sporty, Bohemian, Traditional, Classic, Dramatic,** and **Trendy.**

Let's take a look at each different male type and how they relate in the world.

A SPORTY MAN

Famous Sporty men: Joe Montana, Kurt Russell, John Wayne, Nick Nolte, Prince Andrew, Arnold Schwarzenegger, Bruce Willis

A Sporty man can be found anywhere. While many professional athletes fall into this category, that is not always the case; in fact, there are quite a few who don't. (Note: Don't mistake a Sporty man for a sports fan. They are very different. Any style type except Bohemian can be a sports fan.) Many men in blue-collar jobs are Sporty, because of their dispositions.

A Sporty man does lead an active life. His agility and natural physical strength often land him in strenuous activities. He is happier outdoors and doing anything that keeps him active.

Like the Sporty woman, he is hard on his clothes. While he can dress up and look very elegant, there can sometimes be quite a gap between his jeans and a tux.

Since Sporty men are rarely found in high-level executive positions, suits are simply not a part of his makeup. While he may have a few, they are not a high priority.

Don't misinterpret what I am saying: Sporty men are quite capable of white collar work, it simply is not what makes them happy.

What does he wear?

Like the Sporty woman, this man has a difficult time with anything that is not functional. He prefers to be natural in his clothing and definitely builds his life around being active.

Sporty men do enjoy dressing in fancy suits and tuxedos (mostly for the shock value) since they love to show how good they can really look in a suit. They love looking elegant, but can't wait to get home and get comfortable. Like the Sporty woman, they prefer relaxed functional clothing that makes sense to them.

His life-style is all about convenience and comfort and that is what he'll search out.

Good matches?

A perfect match for a Sporty man is his **Sporty** counterpart. They'll share many common interests, and she won't have a problem with his "lack of polish." She'll love the way her man dresses.

The **Romantic** woman is in for hours of frustration with a man who will appreciate her femininity but not share her need for romance. This is a mismatch, but one that can work if Ms. Romantic is willing to accept that her Sporty man may find pigeon shooting more appealing than a moonlight cruise.

A **Traditional** woman with a Sporty man could appear to be a contradiction. But a Traditional woman can and does adapt well to others, especially her man. Since she so rarely thinks of herself, he may have to drag her shopping from time to time. Their mutual love of children will bond these two together, as will his love of play and her honesty. Their natural abilities combined can create an ideal home environment.

Classic and Sporty can appear to be a mismatch, for here, Sporty will find himself home long before his career-minded mate. She will have to buy him a few outfits for her company dinners, since that is not his forte. He is fairly amicable and will find her world amusing.

However, for harmony to reign here, they will have to live in a place where Sporty can feel comfortable. As long as Classic is given the space to decorate, she can live anywhere. Sporty is happy to let her decorate, as long as there's a comfortable chair in the arrangement. Sporty is very relaxed about his environment, but Ms. Classic cannot function in anything that she feels is not presentable.

Ali McGraw and Steve McQueen were a perfect example of this match.

Whoa. **Dramatic** and Sporty? Yes. While I've never met Dolly Parton's husband Carl, I'm taking a guess that this is their combination. A Dramatic woman needs to be in the limelight, unlike a Sporty man who needs to feel private at times. This can work marvelously since Sporty doesn't begrudge his mate her time in the spotlight.

What about a **Trendy** woman and a Sporty man? One may ask how these two ever got together. Sporty needs consistency and the one thing that he can count on from Trendy is that she will change: her mind, her clothes, and even their home.

However, whenever a Trendy woman marries, if it is to last, it happens because she deems it will. Demi Moore and Bruce Willis are an example of this combination.

Gifts for a Sporty man?

He'll appreciate anything that has to do with his favorite activities. A new glove if he plays softball, camping equipment if he camps, or a new baseball cap with his favorite team insignia on it. If he has children, a day with them doing something active would be heaven.

This is a man to whom functional comfort is important. Always consider that when thinking of what to buy him.

A BOHEMIAN MAN

Famous Bohemian men: James Taylor, Paul McCartney, Lyle Lovett, Jim Morrison, John Lennon, Lenny Kravitz

Like the Romantic woman, this man is driven by his heart. He is so in touch with his feelings that his spouse and he are often extremely close. As much as he may say he wants an equal partner, the Bohemian man can sometimes be surprisingly old-fashioned or even chauvinistic.

This is a man whose family means everything to him. He is very unconventional and probably writes poetry, maybe even does the laundry.

He can be found anywhere from on a farm to a reservation. In general, somewhere that he can be in touch with the land. He is also in love with the idea of natural cooking, and it was probably a Bohemian man who began the first commune. If it was up to him, everyone would live together in peace. Meditation is very likely a part of his routine.

This is not a man who becomes a police officer, because he detests physical violence of any kind. While it is rare to find a Bohemian in a professional position, he may show up as a doctor or an attorney, but only to *really* heal the sick in some Third World country or defend property owned by a minority group being persecuted.

What does he wear?

Since style is the least important thing in his life, clothing is an extremely low priority. Like the Sporty man, his clothes need to be functional; unlike the Sporty man, he needs to feel inspired in his clothes. Bohemian men are frequently nudists, and their having very little clothing isn't necessarily related, they are just minimalists by nature. Communicating his feelings ranks much higher than his appearance.

He may at times have a tousled look, preferring not to spruce himself up to impress anyone. He is not the kind of man who feels appearance counts highly, and consequently he doesn't judge other people by their attire.

His wardrobe can range from surprisingly outdated to unbelievably tacky, but it always works on him. This is a man who is not known for his stylish dress, he is known for his talent.

Don't be surprised to find that he may not own fancy athletic shoes. Expect boots in extreme weather and open-toe sandals the rest of the time.

Good matches?

A Bohemian man, as seemingly sensitive as he is, may want to run the show. If he is so inclined, he will naturally pick a woman who will conform to his style. Or he will let her be the breadwinner, enjoying the household chores and child-rearing process.

As amenable as **Sporty** is, she may tire of a man who's style she feels is too sedentary for her. On the other hand, she could fall head over heels for a man who hikes with her in the wilderness or loves to camp. This match will be determined by the activities they share in common.

Sporty will like his relaxed style of dressing, and his strange wardrobe will not bother her in the least. She may find it necessary to supply him with a pair of athletic shoes to bring him up to par.

The **Romantic** woman is bound to be in love with her man for many lifetimes. The initial attraction here can be quite strong. But, if their interests stray, so can the union. As a team they can be quite memorable. Carly Simon and James Taylor were this combination.

Their home environment will be as warm and inviting as they are. This is one area of total bliss for the two of them, since a Bohemian man will enjoy having his partner run the show.

A **Traditional** woman with a Bohemian man can be quite a peaceful combination. Ms. Traditional will not be bothered by her partner's chauvinistic ways, since she enjoys his love of family and, most of all, her. He will adore her, and she in turn will happily pull the family unit together. Their styles may differ, but his love for her will keep her tendency to be fickle in check.

He will appreciate her style and enjoy her shopping for him.

Of all the style types, the combination of **Classic** woman with a Bohemian man is the least likely. Here is the woman who values career and appearance highly, two things that to a Bohemian man are low priority. His focus is not on his career but on how he can express himself. His waiting for inspiration could drive a Classic nuts since she is constantly on the move.

The problem with this duo is that while he is not style conscious, she is, and if they ever do get past a first date, it could be because he wears a uniform. His lack of refinement in her eyes will soon wear down any feelings she has for him.

However, if a Bohemian can keep the home fires burning while she works and she can buy his clothing, this combo may have a chance.

Dramatic and Bohemian? If Ms. D. perceives his style as outrageous (Mick and Bianca Jagger), then these two can have quite a bit of fun together.

However, when she begins to realize that he really does lack class (in her eyes), and that he doesn't care really what others think of how he looks, that his unkempt appearance is defiance rather than statement, look out. Her need to be adored and loved will soon overpower any love she has left for him when she loses respect for him.

A **Trendy** woman can deal with anyone. But Trendy will demand honesty from her partner, and his need to go inside for answers from his soul may not rest well with her. For Trendy is quick and in some ways impatient, and she will not tolerate anyone who lollygags.

If she perceives for a moment that he is not a team player, she will prod him into it, and he will never really participate. One thing that you can count on is that a Bohemian man is stubborn when he decides he is right, and so is Trendy.

If these two get together it is because Trendy is going through her Bohemian phase and he is attracted to that part of her. As long as their styles stay similar, these two can be blissful.

Gifts for a Bohemian man?

A new journal. A new ink pen. A wild Hawaiian shirt. An outfit that doesn't match. Season tickets to the Philharmonic. Anything that has to do with art or family will appeal to him.

A TRADITIONAL MAN

Famous Traditional Men: Mel Gibson, Martin Luther King, Val Kilmer, Johnny Carson, Garth Brooks, Paul Newman, Billy Crystal, Ron Howard, Jesse Jackson, Tom Hanks

This is a man who understands the meaning of being a partner. His idea of teamwork is sharing with his family. While he does subscribe to the old-fashioned "man as breadwinner" notion, he is also surprisingly respectful and liberated in his own right. He is in many ways the ideal friend and husband. Like his female traditional counterpart, he is a good parent and role model.

No matter what career he chooses, he treats those he works with as family and his loyalty to them is unsurpassed. Most people flock to work with a Traditional man, since his caring and concern never give you the impression that you are anything less than a vital part of the "team."

Even in creative endeavors, these men enjoy working with the same people again and again, creating a safe, fun environment for themselves and others. No matter where he works, you can bet on his loyalty.

The Traditional man tends to have an overdeveloped sense of responsibility toward others, and when stretched too far, it can cause him to overextend himself. For him these things can start honestly enough, but he could find himself disappointing the very people he wanted to help.

What does he wear?

A Traditional man dresses almost exactly like his female Traditional counterpart. Remember that preppie also falls under Traditional, so catalogs like J Crew and L. L. Bean are two examples of catalogs that are unisex and cater to Traditionals.

A Traditional man wears a great deal of what is considered very "American" sportswear. Slacks with a dress shirt (possibly a sport jacket) for casual wear, and suits for dressier occasions.

The era he was born into will dictate a great deal of his wardrobe. And, Traditional, like Sporty and Bohemian, will often have one signature item or piece that they wear that defines them: Ron Howard and his baseball cap, Martin Luther King and his suit.

These men also will rely on their partners or wives to contribute a great deal to their work and life, and hence their accents will vary a great deal depending upon the style type they marry.

Good matches?

Any style type can get along with a Traditional man, for he is truly the ideal partner. Unless he has a dark side that has yet to be uncovered, he is a perfect companion to almost anyone. Each style type will bring a new accent to his life and he will blend well with anyone he is with.

A **Sporty** woman will bring to Mr. Traditional's life a sense of fair play and adventure. Her active life-style will force him into activity that he might not have otherwise enjoyed. These two will share many activities, but Sporty may have to teach him as they go.

In this match up, it may be Traditional who shops for clothes since Sporty is only into the functional side of things. On the other hand, Mr. Traditional will love Sporty's ability to pack up and go with a minimal amount of fuss. A unique combination.

The **Romantic** woman will bring the importance of love and romance into Mr. Traditional's life. She will teach him to see things more gently than he might without her.

He is the perfect man to appreciate her delicate sensibilities, and he will also respect her need for romance. His sensitivity will be heightened by her love of beauty.

Although he will dress in a more traditional vein, he will admire her love of soft fabrics. Romantics love their men to be masculine, so she will like the way he dresses.

A Traditional man has met the perfect match in the **Traditional** woman. Chances are they are similar in almost every way imaginable, and their combined understanding of the importance of putting their friendship first will make for both a solid friendship and mutual respect.

These two will have much to discuss and not surprisingly will enjoy spending a great deal of time with each other and their family.

No matter who shops for clothes, they may share their clothes if their sizes are close, and if not, they quite often wear similar outfits.

Ms. **Classic** too will love her Traditional man, for he will teach her much about family and obligation. She in turn will bring to him the understanding of just how important a role career plays in one's life. She can be the power behind this man, all the while being a creative person in her own right. Her own ambition will spur a fire in her Traditional man.

She will choose to wardrobe him in clothes that she feels will fit his successful image. Therefore, his clothes will become more upscale with her around. Of all the style-type combinations, this is the one that is most noticeable to the Traditional's work colleagues. Before they ever meet her, they know she is the one now choosing his ties and suits, and quite well.

Ms. **Dramatic** will bring much drama to this sedate man's life! She is outspoken and flamboyant and if he respects and admires her beauty these two can be a wonderful mix.

Provided he respects her and can go along with her need to always be in the spotlight, these two can be wonderfully compatible because he understands her deep need to be seen.

She may try to spruce him up, and while he may be pliable in certain areas, he can be just as stubborn as the next man, so she may have to back off where that's concerned. Ernest and Tova Borgnine are this combination.

Since **Trendy** is on the opposite side of the style wheel from Traditional, at first glance it could appear that these two are at odds with one another. But nothing could be farther from the truth. In fact, they borrow many style ideas from one another and can be closer at times than those of the same style type. Mr. Traditional respects this woman for speaking her own mind. He may at times feel intimidated by her ability to open up and say what is on her mind, but he'll be wild about her nonetheless.

Gifts for a Traditional Man?

This man has a strong sense of right and wrong and anything you get him should have some element of that in it. He loves peace and fair play. He would appreciate your gift of sponsoring a child in his name or sending money to his favorite charity. But most of all, he would appreciate time with you (or his children) as a gift. This is a man who doesn't care what he gets, it's the fact that you thought of him. And no matter how goofy the gift, if he loves you, he'll keep it for years.

A CLASSIC MAN

Famous Classic Men: Denzel Washington, Richard Gere, Blair Underwood, John Kennedy, Jr., Ahmad Rashad, Robert Redford, Danny Glover

Here is a man who is unmistakably polished. Even at his most casual, he is well put together. It doesn't hurt the image that Classic men are generally quite handsome, even if they can be self-involved at times. However, once a Classic meets his woman, he is quite easily tamed. He has a sense of style that appeals to most women naturally, and he attracts many people because of his style.

Like his Classic female counterpart, he never appears to be unnerved. He is generally in complete control of a situation, having spent quite a bit of time studying it. He is never a quitter and will pursue whatever he wants until he eventually breaks through. What he lacks in any area, he almost always makes up for in perseverance.

His ability to present himself well in any situation inevitably draws attention to him.

This is a man who will forget anything in pursuit of his career. However, if a woman becomes important in his life, he can pursue her with the same fervor as he would his career. Whatever this man becomes passionate about, he will have.

What does he wear?

The best he can afford to buy is what will find its way into his closet and ultimately onto his body. While he wears labels, he won't wear them because they are labels, per se, he will wear them because that is what he is comfortable in.

This man has a sense of style that is almost inbred, and he can pull together almost anything and look fabulous. From jeans to suits, his is a most complete wardrobe, for he

is comfortable wearing clothes and knows their power.

Good matches?

As wonderful as he is, Mr. Classic can be a loner from time to time, and any woman in his life will have to understand that about him. He is so very dedicated to his career that anyone who doesn't share that with him (or have their own) may find themselves alone quite a bit.

He is a good father, devoted and the like, and if you share that with him, he will consider that a career and be quite steadfast.

A **Sporty** woman may feel at odds with her Classic man from time to time. Although her outdoorsy influence will be great, it may not be enough to pin down a man who's dedication is to his career, not recreation.

He could interpret her love of the outdoors as a call to save the environment and get caught up in a cause of some kind. This is a man who feels a deep need to do something about the injustices in the world, and he and Sporty may share this. Her need to play is a strong one, and she may have to pull him away from his work from time to time in order to get some play time with him!

Their styles are different enough that she will appreciate his sense of style and her ability to pack up and go easily. These two are both very passionate and this can keep home fires burning for quite some time. Cindy Crawford and Richard Gere are this combination.

Mr. Classic will be taken with Ms. **Romantic,** since she can be very elegant and striking. Her passion is about love and romance, though, and it isn't necessarily Mr. Classic's strong suit. She can find herself disappointed if she's waiting for this man to be overly romantic with her.

However, once the Classic man knows what pleases his spouse, he will carry out her wishes with a natural grace. He appreciates her ability to love him so wholeheartedly and, most importantly, just how much she appreciates *him*.

Her love is destined to teach much to this man.

A **Traditional** woman will surprise her Classic partner. Her loyalty to him and their relationship is unsurpassed. She can give him a deep friendship, and he in turn will teach her (if inadvertently) to be more independent. She will have to be a companion to him to keep their relationship vibrant.

Remember that his focus is career and hers is family, and they can easily meld these two styles together.

Classic and Classic are two very busy people. These two lead full lives and for their relationship to work they will each have to make concessions. Continually.

However, they will have a strong attraction to each other's style and share much in common. He will admire the qualities in her that they share, and vice versa. His savoir faire will impress her, and he will enjoy her polish. But most of all, his style of dressing she will most certainly love!

Mr. Classic is ultimately very intimidated by a **Dramatic** woman, and unless he has a very strong personal sense of self, he may not be able to cope with a woman who is as bold and strong as a Dramatic. Theirs is a volatile relationship. Her style often overpowers those she loves, and while it is inadvertent, Classic will not enjoy it in any way.

Their attraction is understandable: hers to a man with polish and drive, not to mention looks; and his to a woman who is flamboyant, bold, and beautiful. But for this to work, she will have to learn to allow him to share, if not have, the spotlight from time to time. A hard feat for Ms. Dramatic to do.

Trendy wants attention when she wants it, and that can create quite a volatile union. Since his focus is career and hers is whatever she feels at the moment, she may want him to share her need for variety, which he may not. He is not intimidated by her, but will have to run to keep up with her.

They are a powerful couple however. Who can forget Demi Moore opposite Robert Redford in *Indecent Proposal?* Their appeal was powerful. And in the movie his character is smitten with her fierce quest for honesty and independence.

Gifts for a Classic Man?

If you know how to shop for his style, he does enjoy clothing. But only if you know his style. This man does end up with quite a few clothing "gifts" that are simply not him.

Something to do with his career would please him. A new briefcase, or a telephone. He loves a gift that has anything to do with what he is passionate about.

A DRAMATIC MAN

Famous Dramatic Men: Arsenio Hall, Eddie Murphy, George Hamilton, Joe Namath, Rob Lowe, Sylvester Stallone, Corbin Bernsen (as Arnie Becker), Fabio

A Dramatic man, like his counterpart, has a very demanding presence. No matter what he does, he loves to have all eyes on him. He can be outrageous and can easily intimidate others. If his success has gone to his head, he can be quite arrogant. If not, he loves to be benevolent to others and can be amazingly kind. His gutsy style is part of what makes him popular.

He enjoys attention and knows how to gain yours. From humor to his looks, this man is acutely aware of the qualities he possesses that are outstanding, and he isn't shy about revealing them.

Many Dramatic men are thought to have huge egos. Perhaps it's their overdeveloped confidence. They are not necessarily the marrying kind. Why? Because they have trouble sharing attention with another person. However, if they do fall (and stay) in love, they can be quite devoted, especially if their spouse is as devoted to them.

Everything this man does he does in a big way, and his generosity is no different. When he is magnanimous, the world will know it, for he does have trouble keeping his good deeds to himself.

What does he wear?

His appearance has a great deal to do with a Dramatic man's makeup. Although his clothing choices are hardly outrageous, they are not understated. He is not afraid of wearing clothing by the finest designers, and revels in his own ability to do so.

He will wear anything that he feels is elegant. This is a man to whom clothing means a great deal. He is an impeccable dresser and will want his woman to draw the same attention to him that his clothing does. For anything he surrounds himself with is destined to be a head turner. That simply is his style.

Consider too that even bodybuilding can be something a Dramatic man gets into, since that would attract attention to him. With a Dramatic man, power is everything.

He is not afraid of being controversial in his romantic choices and may surprise many with whom he chooses. If he's controversial, he's Dramatic.

Good matches?

Any woman who finds herself with a Dramatic man must adore him. Perhaps more than any other man, this is something he craves and needs to have in order to stay with a mate. While many crave the attention in the beginning of a relationship, it is something that changes over time as people get to know one another. Not for Mr. Dramatic, who will continue to need the same attention that was given to him at the beginning. If you choose a Dramatic man, you are in for entertainment, for he is certainly charming.

A **Sporty** woman may wonder what all the fuss is about. These two can be quite compatible if his focus is his body or sports in any way. Quite a few Dramatic athletes marry Sporty women since they are so active. And, because Sporty is so supportive (always the coach/ cheerleader), a Dramatic man will find her very appealing. Sporty is inner directed and in touch with herself, unlike Mr. Dramatic, who is more concerned with how others

perceive him, so she can be wonderfully grounded for him. If he can bear it.

Dramatic will want a home environment that is far more showy than what Sporty likes; she only desires a place to hang her hat. If their home resembles a fancy hunting lodge or ski house, then Sporty is easily appeased and Dramatic can show it off to his friends and associates.

When a **Romantic** woman meets Mr. Dramatic, her love for him and his need for her love can keep them afloat for a while. But alas, under Dramatic's show there is not always the substance to make a relationship last, unlike a Romantic woman, who can stay in love for many years, long after a relationship has ended, in fact.

Unfortunately what I've seen happen in this combination is that Ms. Romantic will support (or be supportive) of Mr. Dramatic during his rise, and once he has risen, he won't "love" her anymore.

On the other hand, if she's working and developing on her own, then it is possible for this union to work. Just remember that Mr. D thrives on attention. Without it, he will drift.

A **Traditional** woman is often quite well suited to a Dramatic man, for she can and will handle all the things he won't wish to. A Traditional woman is a perfect detail person, while Mr. Dramatic enjoys the results. Unfortunately she, like her Romantic sister, is in danger of being left by this man once success strikes him.

He is flamboyant and that may attract her to him, but unfortunately, she may never get the deep love she craves from this man, for he may not be capable of giving it.

Of all men, Dramatic men may stray.

The **Classic** woman may have a hard time with a man, who is more flashy than she is. This is one woman who will resent his pontificating. It will annoy her. She won't appreciate his being at the mirror more than she.

This is a woman who appreciates fine things but would never feel comfortable flaunting them. Such is the problem with this combination: he'll show, she'll hide.

For this to work, Mr. Dramatic will have to slow down and share the limelight with his mate, and she will have to appreciate his dramatic nature.

A **Dramatic**/Dramatic combination is definitely sink or swim! These are two distinct personalities that could never just "get along okay." This is either perfect or a horrible mismatch. Brigitte Nielsen and Sylvester Stallone were both Dramatics.

Since they both attract considerable attention, this can be quite a powerful combination. Privately, they will have to work at sharing much more than just their love of attention, although sexual compatibility can keep these two dancing for quite a long time.

A Dramatic man will enjoy a spouse as radiant as he feels he is, and they could be a popular couple, involved in activities and in the community.

Ms. **Trendy** will definitely keep Mr. Dramatic on his toes. Not a woman to take any flack, she will demand equal attention and an equal partner. A Dramatic man will stand in awe of a woman who can so powerfully influence his life by just being in it. Her no-nonsense approach will be very appealing to him, and he will adore her at the same time he is slightly intimidated by her.

Gifts for a Dramatic Man?

Since appearance is quite important to him, personal grooming products go over well with a Dramatic man. Anything that draws attention to him in a positive way is also perfect for him.

If you do buy clothing for him, don't take it personally if he returns it for something slightly more flashy. He is very hard to shop for. Consider yourself skilled if you know how to shop for a Dramatic man.

A TRENDY MAN

Famous Trendy Men: Spike Lee, Jack Nicholson, Elvis Presley, Bruce Lee, Sam Shepard, Graham Greene, Dwight Yoakam, Tim Robbins, Al Pacino, James Dean

The most important information to relay about a Trendy man is that no matter what, he never ever follows any trend. He is the trendsetter, the man who sets his own style and has his own way of doing things. A Trendy man is a man who does things in his own way.

This man is not afraid to stand his ground no matter what. He can also surprise you by giving up when he's just about to win because he decides that it doesn't matter to him anymore. He may be fickle at times, but this is a man who truly knows what he wants. Professionally he'll challenge himself constantly, always willing to do whatever he feels compelled to do. In fact, he revels in going against the "norm" or what is socially acceptable.

He is a man with many, many facets to his personality. Just when you think him a confirmed bachelor, he'll turn around and propose. He really doesn't care for outside opinions; although he will consider them, he doesn't live by them.

Those close to him have a strong influence on him, and he can love quite deeply, but he might not want to live the way others prescribe for him.

This man is, in a word, *unconventional*. This trait is not something he works at or aspires to, it simply is who he is. His honesty does at times get him into trouble, but there is one definite with him: integrity. He is sincere and it is not in his nature to mislead anyone. While people can and do get mislead by his actions, it is not of his doing. Others tend to see what they want to regarding him.

To be a part of this man's life, you must accept him as he is or don't even bother.

What Does He Wear?

Trendy can show up wearing whatever his current whim reflects. If it's high fashion, he won't necessarily care to wear it. Only if it suits his present mood. He is influenced by those around him and his environment very strongly, and if moved enough, he could drastically change his style overnight.

Since he can show up wearing anything at any time, he is the man who is most changeable, and hence most accepting of whatever you wear.

What he definitely won't wear is the designer of the moment (unless of course, it suits him).

Good matches?

Whew! This is one man who is difficult to pin down. Trendy men can range from too possessive to uncaring. He is not the image of the perfect family man, unless he feels it's what he wants, but even still he's not really for the long haul. Not because he's not capable, but the truth is that Trendy men tend to be as unpredictable as their style. Therefore, there is no way to tell you exactly what to expect from a Trendy man.

In general, problems occur with a Trendy man when you would like him to do something your way. This is a man to whom marriage and commitment have to come on his own terms and in his own way, and even then they may be slightly unconventional. The fact is that this man is so unpredictable, it's hard to predict what a relationship with a different style type could actually be like since so much of it depends upon him. But I'll try.

A **Sporty** woman contains all the qualities that Mr. Trendy would admire, especially since she is ahead of him on the style wheel. But she would have to be fiercely independent to keep this man in her life.

This match is as unable to predict as Trendy himself is.

A **Romantic** woman will get to do a great deal of pining with a Trendy man, for he may not be around very much. This man does change course like the wind, and while he may never make any proclamations of undying love, he could easily break Romantic's heart with his tendency toward callousness.

Romantic will wait for a while, but once burned, she'll never return to him. On the other hand, this combination can work marvelously if she is willing to accept her relationship with this man on his terms, and of all the style types, she's the one who could. She is a wonderful power-behind-the-throne type, and she could make herself so valuable to him that without her he is helpless.

A **Traditional** woman will be instantly smitten with her Trendy man. She will enjoy his wild side. She will either nurture it and grow with him, or he will grow away from her. If he grows away from her, she will begin to resent all his fun wild qualities that once drew her to him.

She may possess the consistency that he craves, and if that is the case this can be a wonderful union. She will also support him in his endeavors—and while he broods.

In the case of a **Classic** woman, this is definitely oil and water. The up side to this, of course, is that she can easily stand up to him! Ms. Classic is not the woman to sit at home and pine over anyone. Since she's a career woman, she'll always be able to run off and take care of herself, and that is something that she may have to do if she gets involved with a Trendy man.

However, this could be a fun mix because Mr. T is intrigued with women who do their own thing.

Trouble lies ahead for Mr. Trendy if he crosses a **Dramatic** woman. She is not easily amused by his anecdotes and could be embarrassed by his lack of savoir faire in public.

He truly does not run his clock based upon what others think and that can definitely drive Ms. D right over the edge. She cares too much about her appearance to be with a man who has nothing to prove and doesn't.

A **Trendy** woman with her counterpart can be a wonderful combination. She understands on a very deep level his need to make himself over every once in a while and in addition his need to be his own person. Her constantly changing before his eyes will keep him interested and searching at home for new adventures. Yes, being with a woman as un-

predictable as he is could be the perfect match for Mr. Trendy.

Gifts for a Trendy Man?

What can you get for a man who is in constant transition? If Trendy has a consistent interest, you may try that first. If he likes football or basketball, season tickets or a T-shirt would be nice. He does love the unusual, so surprising him with something out of the ordinary could prove quite interesting.

Remember the original quiz? The typical Trendy answer about the free trip would be to go wherever they felt like it at the moment. See what his interests are at the moment and buy him something related to them. The key is not to buy anything too far in advance. Because guaranteed, it won't be long before he's off doing something else!

Chapter Twelve

CLEARING OUT YOUR CLOSET

There are always three dominant colors for each woman. The first color (what *you* love to wear) is the way that you see yourself. Yellow, for instance, may indicate that you see yourself as a real "team" player, someone who gets along well with others, has a positive attitude, and is quite rational. This color may change over time, as you do, but it generally is a color you will always own.

The second color is the color you get the most compliments on. It reflects how others see you. For instance, if red is the color you receive the most compliments on, the world may see you as a more "self-oriented" person. You can look up your particular shade or hue in the glossary and gain valuable insights into yourself.

And finally, your power color is the one you feel the most confident in. If you choose purple, for example, you may derive your confidence for being above the crowd rather than a part of it. You may be feel best when you are in total control without someone else telling you what to do.

These colors are the ones to keep an eye on as you clear out your closet, for they will be the basis around which to frame a functional wardrobe.

THE DARK ROOM

Now, going through your closet may be a traumatic experience. If it's any consolation (I know it's not) I've had closet trauma and survived. Do yourself a service and take the time to do it right. You won't want to do it again for quite a while, and if you do it thoroughly you won't have to.

Here's my suggested procedure:

• As you look through the clothes in your closet, imagine each article on another woman who has the same style as you do. If you can't think of anyone, you can use the examples I've provided for you in the beginning of your style chapter.
• If a garment does not fit into your style and you have not worn it for at least a year, give it away.
• If, however, the outfit *is* your style, but you're still not wearing it, here's another option: put any questionable items in a box to store for a season. If after that season you don't miss them, it may be time to part.
• Definitely rid yourself of *anything* that you haven't worn in at least two seasons (say, two winters in a row).
• Remove all "somedays"—items that do not currently fit your body. I can't tell you how much weight I lost when I finally got rid of those pants that I was going to someday lose enough weight to fit into.

> **Tip:** If your "current" size bothers you, cut out your size tags.
>
> **Tip:** Every closet should have an easy "fat day" outfit that looks great on you and is marvelously loose and comfortable!

• Remove all style clashes. You may have had a sporty feeling at Nordstrom's fall sale; however, if you're really a Classic, it may be time to create more room for your style.

> **Tip:** Have a clothes swapping party and organize each section by "style" type. This way your Romantic friend can get that frilly blouse you never wear, and you can acquire a catsuit from your Sporty friend who never wears it.
>
> **Tip:** Throw out or give away *any* pieces that are too small for you! Unless you are presently losing weight, stop torturing yourself with those items that fit years ago. When a client accidentally bought a pair of jeans that were one size too large for her, I told her to keep them. She reported to me that she always feels fantastic in them! She realized that she began to eat more sensibly every time she put them on because her size wasn't a big deal anymore. She's lost one full dress size since then.

If you love a particular outfit and can't figure out how to wear it, it's probably because it's not quite your style. You may have to pull it apart and add something in your style type to change the focal point of the outfit; using accessories is one way to achieve this. The main thing is to remove items that are simply not you.

• Now hang all the remaining clothes in *color order*. Begin with white and progress to black. First yellow or beige then peach or pink through greens, blues, reds, purples, browns, grays, and blacks. This is another way to find the colors you are most often complimented on, as well as attracted to. Don't be surprised to see a quite a bit of your three personal colors when you begin to sort out your wardrobe. Most women tend to buy more things in their personal colors.

The benefit to this is, of course, that you get to see how much clothing you already own that is workable for you and at the same time see the many different combinations for your personal colors. This will give you new ways to wear your clothing.

> **Tip:** Years ago, women could easily find *their* colors in their actual season. Today manufacturers have gotten wise to this, and since they want you to shop year-round, they are mixing seasons and you'll be able to find all the "seasonal" colors year-round. Keep in mind that you will still find more of the cool winter colors in winter and warm spring colors in spring.

- Notice if the remaining colors in your closet work together so that you will have complete outfits left. For example, a peach skirt might not fit anymore, but the matching blazer will work with your white skirt. Get out a pad of paper and begin to make your shopping list; write down any piece you feel will complete your current wardrobe.

Do not edit your list! Write everything down. You may not feel that you really need it at this point, but you should list it anyway. Put this list aside, and let's do accessories. We'll come back to this in a minute.

> **Tip:** Often new seasonal colors are simply new color combinations and not new colors entirely. While everyone might be wearing red and green one season, it'll be red and hot pink the next. So if you keep abreast of the "in" combinations, that will help keep you current without having to spend a fortune updating your wardrobe.

TAKING INVENTORY OF YOUR ACCESSORIES

- Take out *all* of your accessories—hats, handbags, scarves, belts, jewelry, panty hose, and shoes—and lay them out so you can see them. A bed, table, or football field will do.
- Remove things that are broken, worn out (add these items to your shopping list), somedays (too big or too small), riddled with painful memories, or that you just don't like anymore.
- Do the accessories you have now work with what you have left in your closet? What do you need to add, anything?

- Do you have any "fantasy" accessories? A special watch or belt that you won't buy because it wouldn't "work for you"? Or is too expensive? Write those down on your list.
- Do the same thing with accessories that you did with your clothing. Ask yourself, "Is this my style?" If it isn't you, get rid of it (unless it's a family heirloom, those are keepers no matter what).

ASSESSING YOUR NEEDS

Now that you've made up a list, it's time to assess your needs. We'll need to determine whether each item on your list is of primary or secondary importance. Before you do that, I have one suggestion: flip to your style chapter and compare your list with the *basics* listed there. If there are *any* matches, that item is a primary for you.

Now next to each item on your list, put a small *p* or *s* (for primary and secondary). Next, separate out the two lists. Don't forget to note the color you'd like each item in if that's important to you.

Your primary list is comprised of items that you must be willing to pay full price for, if necessary. No guilt allowed. These are pieces you need in order to fill out your wardrobe. They are vital and you will wear them for a long

time. They are what I call investments. This is "investment dressing."

Your second list is of less importance, and you may not be willing to pay full price for those items. Nor should you. These are whim pieces, things that will add but not "make" your wardrobe. If there is anything on this list that you cannot live without, remove it and put it on the primary list.

Next to each thing on *both* lists, write down the amount of money you are willing to pay for each item. This is your spending plan, so no cheating allowed. Be fair to yourself. Don't underestimate the cost or you'll be setting yourself up for disappointment. I always try to overestimate on my spending plan. Here's a perfect example of what I mean:

I have a Trendy client who already owns three black skirts, one in leather, another in wool, and the third in linen. So as you can see, she really doesn't *need* another one. But she wanted one, so she put a sheer black skirt on her secondary list. She then planned $75.00 for it.

One day, she stumbled across a sheer black skirt on sale while visiting a very traditional city. It was a famous designer skirt on a final markdown rack. It was $30.00. Was it worth it? You bet! Besides, it was her secondary list and less than her spending plan. This allowed her to buy a jacket for which she had underestimated the cost that was on her primary plan! Hence, no guilt!

Do be reasonable in your choices. Don't be so specific that you set yourself up for disappointment.

When I do seminars in department stores, I'm amazed by just how overly specific women can be about what they want. One day a woman came up to me after a seminar and described in great detail a dress she was looking for.

I was standing next to the dress department manager, and she asked the customer where she'd had seen this dress.

The customer said that she hadn't seen it, but it was what she wanted. I looked at her and teased, "You mean you've never seen this dress. You don't know if it exists. It's simply a picture in your head, but you'd like us to show it to you?" At this point the woman herself began to laugh.

I lightly told her that she wouldn't like anything we showed her because it wouldn't live up to her fantasy dress.

She agreed with me.

I asked her if she was willing to try something that *did* exist.

She was and I showed her a traditional dress. She bought it. It was completely different than what she originally had asked for. It also happened that she was a Traditional and was searching for a Classic. When I showed her a traditional dress, it made sense to her.

My point? She was happy when she let go of her fantasy of being a Classic and began dressing in her own style.

This is the problem with just buying to create an effect you want rather than buying the correct style. When I give seminars, it's not uncommon for a woman that I worked with a year ago to come up to me wearing what I told her to buy last year.

This happened to me on a trip to Columbia, South Carolina, not too long ago. A customer came up to me and, pointing to the sweater she was wearing, reminded me that I had told her the year before that it was so perfect for her, I wouldn't let her leave the store without it. I was somewhat embarrassed. "I guess I can be outspoken at times," I said.

"Oh, no," she responded. "This was the best purchase I ever made. Can you tell me what else I need?"

What she needed was to keep buying things that were the correct style type for her. The items we buy that we felt we'd paid too much for at the time but wear forever are the things that are our style type. Choose more hits.

Spend the money for clothes that are the correct style type and you'll have a wardrobe that you're proud of. Now that you have your list, let's talk a moment about money.

MONEY

The very first thing to remember when you go to buy clothes is that you are making an investment in you. I always suggest you spend more money on an everyday item that you will wear frequently than on an item you'll wear once.

Many women get sticker shock from the price of clothing. One way to take the sting out of spending is to consider what the *cost per wearing* of the outfit you are buying will be.

Consider this: A jacket you want is $350. You figure out that you'll wear it 5 times a month. Multiply the 5 by 12 months (it usually evens out, since you may wear it more some months than others) which equals 60. Now, divide 350 by 70. $5.80.

That's what your new jacket will cost per wearing in the first year. Consider, too, that it will be even less expensive as the years pass.

Cost per wearing on a $250 dress? Let's say you'll wear it twice a month for a year. Divide 24 into 250. That comes to approximately $10.00 per wearing for the *first* year. Again, if you wear it for two years, slice the price in half; for three years, in thirds, and so on.

For formal wear, divide the price by 5 years, then again by the amount of times you'll wear it per year. That will be your cost per wearing. If the price is $350, for example, divided by 5 is $70. Divide again by 3 and your approximate cost per wearing is $23.33.

Keep in mind that there are many pieces we buy that wind up costing far less and they offset the more expensive items. Sportswear, for example, works out to less because the pieces are separate and can be worn more frequently.

But that doesn't mean that sportswear is the best purchase all the time.

WHEN TO SPEND MORE AND WHEN NOT TO

Don't be afraid of spending too much on a suit or outstanding jacket. Good quality will last a long time. In addition, you can save on blouses or on shoes on sale.

You don't always have to spend more on leggings, turtlenecks, or shorts. Those items can always be gotten for less. Most of the time we have to replace summer items since they wear out faster.

HOW TO SET UP A BUYING PLAN

I have one more suggestion regarding the amount of money you spend on your clothes.

Five percent. That's right. Five percent. If you set up a savings account and put in 5 percent of your earnings, you will have an appropriate percentage to spend on your clothes. Some women will spend more, some less, so use this as a general guide to judge what is necessary for you.

Now, take out your shopping list. Add up the figures on the list, and you will have a rough idea of the amount in your spending plan.

The good thing about putting money aside in a savings account is it reduces the guilt we feel when we shop. I'm always amazed how many women buy something, then qualify their purchase with, "Well, I guess I need it."

Being prepared is also wonderful because you don't have to put your purchases on credit cards. Ouch! We almost never pay the credit off all at once, and then we're playing catch up with payments! So, saving up and being prepared is a viable alternative.

Now that you have your list and your spending plan, you're ready for the next section of the book, "Using Color with Your Style."

In the next chapter I've provided a color and style wheel for each season. Chances are your three "personal" colors are on one of the color wheels. If you use them as a guide, they will assist you in matching colors that will build and expand your wardrobe.

SECTION II

USING COLOR
WITH YOUR STYLE

Chapter Thirteen

SEASONAL COLOR AND STYLE WHEELS

Years ago the theory was that you needed to buy only neutrals and then build your wardrobe around them. Then along came the seasonal color theory, telling women that they could use color, but just the right ones.

Yet even with all this change, many fashion books suggest using neutrals to build a wardrobe. This idea works if you're a Traditional (sometimes a Sporty or a Classic). But it doesn't necessarily hold true for the other style types.

Ms. Trendy, for example, may think of purple as her "neutral," the color with which all others in her closet must coexist. This isn't to say that neutrals don't work, it's simply that we don't have to hold to that idea if it doesn't work for us.

Besides, most women are not starting with nothing. Most of us already have a ward-

robe, and somehow we've managed all these years to find "something" to wear. That means there is a wardrobe in the middle of all those clothes, and now through knowing your personal style, it's emerging.

I've designed the four seasonal color wheels to work within the original style wheel.

You'll notice the "home" color of your style will always remain the same. On the next page is an illustration of the style wheel with color added. You'll see that I've broken color into six groups, beginning with the active red and moving up to the more free purple.

Each of the style types brings a different aspect of their style to a particular color. Accenting with color is inherently powerful, especially if it falls on your seasonal palette.

The design of these wheels is to help you look at the colors of your palette in a different

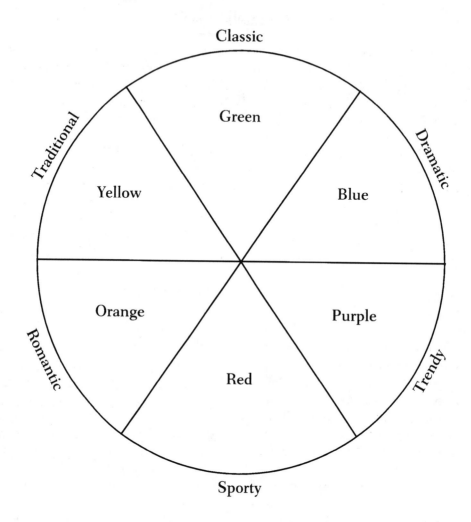

The Style/Color Wheel

way. You may find that your "power" color or your "compliment" color falls into the section where your accent style type resides.

Another aspect of these wheels is that most of the colors on your wheel work easily together. However, if you borrow colors from another palette, then you may need to pay special attention to matching colors. Remember: if you borrow a color from another palette, it might not blend easily with what is already in your closet. Borrow wisely.

Let's take a look at each of the six style and color categories before going to your wheel.

Sporty/Red

Starting things is easy for a Sporty, and such is the energy of red, which symbolizes the beginning or fire underneath everything. This is always the blessing/curse of being a Sporty. She is fabulous at getting things started; on the flip side, she tends to run on to the next thing before completing the last. It's organization and follow-through that can take some effort on her part.

Romantic/Orange

The energy of orange is movement and emotions (in relation to sex and intimacy). Romantic, who is driven by love, finds her match with orange. This can create an all or nothing problem in her life, for if there is no love, she feels like nothing. Hence the cycle of being a romantic style type.

Traditional/Yellow

The ability to rationalize and think things through is found in yellow. It is also the cooperation color and denotes a "team player." This color lands in the traditional area for a reason! On the flip side for Ms. Traditional, she may run the risk of losing her individuality for "the good of the whole."

Classic/Green

Since green pertains to matters of the heart, or feeling emotionally connected, it would stand to reason that we often find Classics doing whatever they feel passionate about. At the same time, it becomes easy to understand why Ms. Classic tends to lose her perspective when she is emotionally involved with something or someone.

Dramatic/Blue

The color of communication, blue echoes Ms. Dramatic's need to be *heard*. She communicates her message every time she appears, sometimes fairly strongly. The obvious thing here is that she does communicate, just that sometimes it's too much.

Trendy/Purple

Purple is associated with spirituality as well as royalty. This is one woman who does not need to sit in a loincloth to be spiritual! She lives her life in a spiritual way, no matter how she earns her living, and there is a sincerity and purity to her style.

Trendy naturally has the majestic quality associated with purple. She is regal in her ability to be herself, always.

COLOR AND STYLE

The seasonal color theories are fabulous and a wonderful starting point for color usage. A color palette takes at most a few hours to have done. But there may be additional colors that work for you that aren't always determined by a quick appointment with a color analyst.

The idea behind the seasonal color theory was to help expand what a woman's color choices were, not limit them. I'm a spring coloration, but accents from the autumn palate work wonderfully for me. This is why I believe

it's important to learn the rules of a system, then break them.

Many of you probably know your "season" already. Aside from having your colors professionally done, there are three other clues to finding your season. Consider the following questions:

1. What is your favorite season—winter, spring, summer, or autumn?
2. What climate do you prefer, cold or warm?
3. On what seasonal palette do at least two of your three colors fall? (Don't count black if it's your power color, since that only falls on the winter chart. You'll have to use your other two colors. If they are on two different seasonal charts, consider if they're warm or cool, then look at the balance of your wardrobe, which chart do most of your colors fall on?)

Frequently, our favorite season tends to be our seasonal color.

I have a client who hates heat! Give her cold weather any day. She also happens to be a winter. Summers too tend to like cooler weather, they live in air-conditioning. While springs and autumns gravitate more to warmer climates.

Obviously, if you locate your personal colors on one palette, this is another clue to uncovering your season.

When I'm working with a client, sometimes I'll use the slice of the wheel that represents her style type to build out from colorwise. For example, if I'm working with a Romantic, and she's a spring or autumn, then I'll begin in the orange family. If she's a winter or summer, I'll begin with the colors that oppose her on the wheel, like the cool blues that fall into the Dramatic's quadrant.

And finally, there is one more element to these wheels: notice where your type falls and what the natural colors are in your quadrant.

A friend of mine who is a winter called me up one evening. She was concerned that I had overlooked something on the basic color wheel for her. She informed me that I must have made a mistake because there were no colors in the orange quadrant of the winter wheel.

I remarked that I'd never seen her wear orange.

She didn't, but she wanted to just let me know that it was missing. Then she tried to ask without asking what that meant, if a color wasn't represented on your wheel.

It really just means that those aren't the colors of your season. Typically, the qualities that are associated with a missing color are already ingrained in the personality. There are times when it could be an imbalance, but that is something that an individual has to decide for themselves.

The idea is to study your individual wheel and notice where you fall on it. Then, develop your wardrobe based on the colors that work best with your personal style. The seasonal wheels are on pages 175–178.

Have fun!

SPRING

The first seasonal wheel contains the colors of springtime blossoms. The neutrals for this wheel are: brown, honey, light gray, gold and ivory, spring's "white."

You borrow most easily from autumn's warm colors, and especially the colors in your style type quadrant of another seasonal wheel.

AUTUMN

The crisp feel of the air as the leaves change, a time when nature prepares for her winter respite. If you are in this seasonal palette, welcome! The autumn seasonal wheel contains the warm colors of the fall season. The neutrals for this block are: brown, camel, olive, rust. Ivory is autumn's "white" for this season. You borrow most easily from spring's warm colors, and especially the colors in your style type quadrant of another seasonal wheel.

WINTER

The winter seasonal wheel contains the cool colors of winter. The neutrals for this season are: all grays, black, taupe, greige, navy, silver, and white. If you recognize your personal colors here, then this is your wheel. Remember it is easier to borrow from the cool summer wheel than any other palette. You can also borrow the colors in your style type quadrant of another seasonal wheel.

SUMMER

The summer seasonal wheel contains the cool colors of summer. The neutrals for this sea-son are: gray, tan, rich cranberry, navy, taupe, cocoa, and off-white. If you recognize your personal colors here, then this is your wheel. Borrow from the cool winter wheel before any other. You can also borrow the colors in your style type quadrant of another seasonal wheel.

Now you've got style, you've got color . . .

. . . but what would happen if you want to convey a statement at work, for example, and knew the color that supported your point of view? Your communication would become more powerful. On the same note, if you want to play down an aspect of your personality, you can do it with color.

In the next chapter, you'll find the meanings of the colors you already wear and some you may want to add!

Next up . . .

the color glossary.

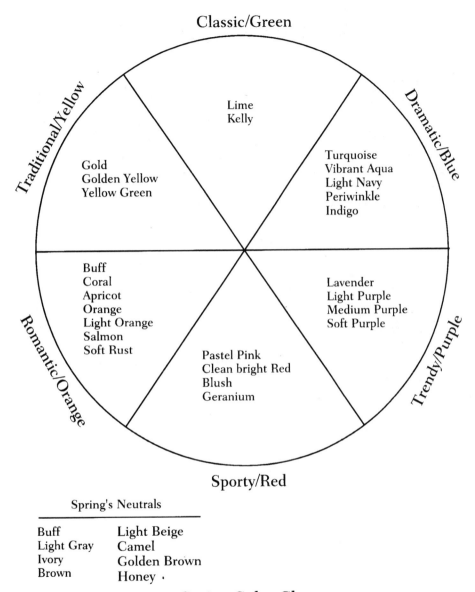

Classic/Green

Lime
Kelly

Dramatic/Blue

Turquoise
Vibrant Aqua
Light Navy
Periwinkle
Indigo

Traditional/Yellow

Gold
Golden Yellow
Yellow Green

Buff
Coral
Apricot
Orange
Light Orange
Salmon
Soft Rust

Lavender
Light Purple
Medium Purple
Soft Purple

Trendy/Purple

Romantic/Orange

Pastel Pink
Clean bright Red
Blush
Geranium

Sporty/Red

Spring's Neutrals

Buff	Light Beige
Light Gray	Camel
Ivory	Golden Brown
Brown	Honey ·

Spring Color Chart

1 7 5

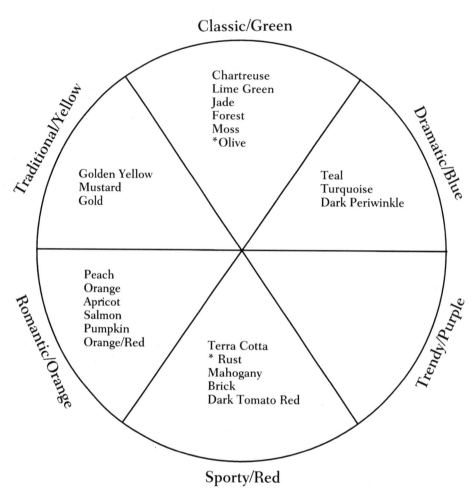

Classic/Green

Chartreuse
Lime Green
Jade
Forest
Moss
*Olive

Traditional/Yellow

Dramatic/Blue

Golden Yellow
Mustard
Gold

Teal
Turquoise
Dark Periwinkle

Peach
Orange
Apricot
Salmon
Pumpkin
Orange/Red

Romantic/Orange

Trendy/Purple

Terra Cotta
* Rust
Mahogany
Brick
Dark Tomato Red

Sporty/Red

Autumn's Neutrals

Oyster	Chocolate Brown
Brown	Greige
Camel	All Beiges
Bronze	*Rust
Coffee	*Olive

Autumn Color Chart

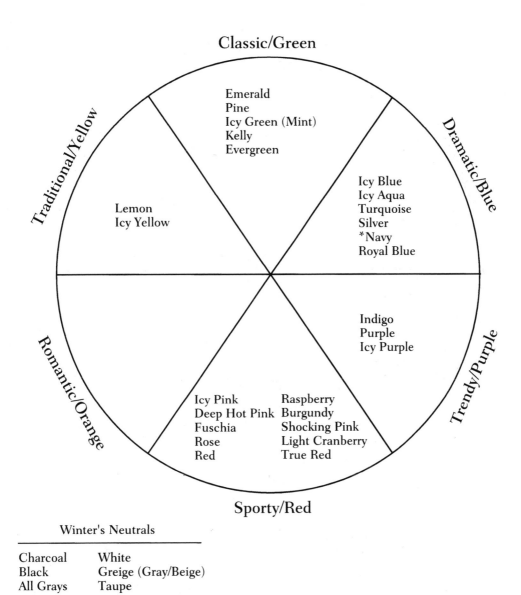

Classic/Green

Emerald
Pine
Icy Green (Mint)
Kelly
Evergreen

Traditional/Yellow

Dramatic/Blue

Lemon
Icy Yellow

Icy Blue
Icy Aqua
Turquoise
Silver
*Navy
Royal Blue

Indigo
Purple
Icy Purple

Romantic/Orange

Trendy/Purple

Icy Pink   Raspberry
Deep Hot Pink Burgundy
Fuschia   Shocking Pink
Rose   Light Cranberry
Red   True Red

Sporty/Red

Winter's Neutrals

Charcoal   White
Black   Greige (Gray/Beige)
All Grays   Taupe

Winter Color Chart

177

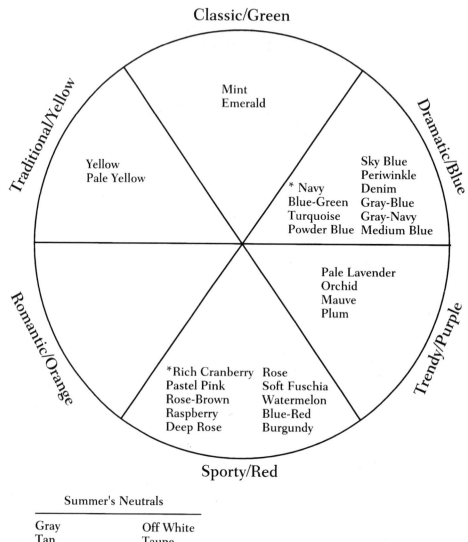

Classic/Green

Traditional/Yellow

Dramatic/Blue

Mint
Emerald

Yellow
Pale Yellow

Sky Blue
Periwinkle
Denim
Gray-Blue
Gray-Navy
Medium Blue

* Navy
Blue-Green
Turquoise
Powder Blue

Pale Lavender
Orchid
Mauve
Plum

Trendy/Purple

Romantic/Orange

*Rich Cranberry
Pastel Pink
Rose-Brown
Raspberry
Deep Rose

Rose
Soft Fuschia
Watermelon
Blue-Red
Burgundy

Sporty/Red

Summer's Neutrals

Gray	Off White
Tan	Taupe
*Rich Cranberry	Cocoa
*Navy	

Summer Color Chart

1 7 8

Chapter Fourteen

COLOR GLOSSARY

Each color emanates a particular energy. Here is a quick key to each solid color; in the glossary below you'll find many of the shades and hues of these color families.

Neutrals
Neutrals are: black, white, gray, taupe, greige (gray-beige)
Neutrals say: "I will make little or no statement. That is up to you."
Overall Impression: anonymity

Red
Red: vital, sexual, passionate, energized, forceful
Red says: "I am self motivated from the center of my being."
Gem: ruby
Overall impression: passion

Orange
Orange: activity, motivator, optimistic, courage, sociable, enthusiasm, affection, humanitarian
Orange says: "If you follow me, I can inspire you and countless others."
Gem: pearls
Overall impression: warmth

Yellow
Yellow: creative, intelligent, precise, cooperative, reasonable, innovation, originality, wisdom
Yellow says: "Intellect is everything."
Gem: coral
Overall impression: rational

Green

Green: balance, harmony, brotherhood, hope, growth, healing, love, peace, prosperity

Green says: "With proper balance, anything is possible."

Gem: emerald

Overall impression: sensual

Blue

Blue: truth, communication, loyalty, serenity, faith, spirituality, creativity, expression

Blue says: "I will allow you to see the truth through me."

Gem: moonstones

Overall impression: communication

Purple

Purple: intuitive, spiritual, royalty, respected, distinguished, proud, aloof, humble, creative imagination

Purple says: "I live in a world of beauty and imagination. If you choose to join me, please wipe your feet before entering."

Gem: sapphire

Overall impression: creative imagination

COLOR GLOSSARY

The following is a glossary of colors. If you don't find the color you are looking for, try another name. Some of the colors are so close that they may carry the same meaning.

Amethyst

Amethyst gives off the very powerful message that you are unwavering. Wear amethyst when you need to concentrate intensely on your work.

It is not the color to wear when you are going to have to alter your work to another's specifications, nor should you wear it when you are on a team project. It gives the impression that no matter what, you are capable of completing any task.

This is a highly spiritual color that radiates confidence and self-expression in the most positive of ways. Much healing happens around amethyst. It is a wonderful, purifying color.

Apple (Granny Smith Green)

The mixture of yellow and green combine to make apple. Wearing apple tells others that you have an innate curiosity about everything, but you cannot be pinned down! People seeking adventure will follow you when you wear apple. Your free spirit will get projects started, but apple may not be the best color to instill confidence in your ability to follow through. While your heart may be in the start-up, apple warns that you may not be able to do the tedious detail work.

Apple is a wonderful color to wear when brainstorming ideas, or in the development stages of something. Everyone wants to be associated with excitement, and with apple you will deliver, people will be attracted to your open-minded approach to whatever you are doing.

Whether or not you wear apple to a job interview depends greatly upon the job you are applying for. My Trendy client Gina wore an apple-colored suit on an interview for a job she was later offered. Of course, being creative director at an ad agency fits the energy of apple perfectly!

Apricot

Apricot is the color of the lone wolf, the most aloof of the orange family. It indicates to others that while you are friendly and available, you are quite content being by yourself. Apricot tends to bring out the contemplative side to anyone who wears it.

Apricot is a wonderful weekend color because it is very relaxing. It's great for a picnic, for example, because it tells others that you are organized, yet able to have fun. It highlights your organization skills (packing a picnic basket), as well as creating energy to play and have fun.

Volunteer work is wonderfully matched to apricot, for it tells others that you willingly would do whatever needs to get done.

Wear apricot when you wish to get things done in a quiet, unobtrusive way.

Aqua

Aqua tells the observer that you are true to yourself, even if you are sometimes overly idealistic. Wearing aqua conveys an aura of trustworthiness. While truth is an important element of any tone of blue, you are not governed by your intellect, but from a deeper sense of propriety: what "feels" right to you.

Baby Blue

The beginning blue is found here. It is the color of hopeful imagination. It signifies creativity and beginning. Others perceive you as being able to be quite analytical when need be, yet imaginative in your problem solving. While blue is typically honest (blue is "true blue"), you are very creative in the way you deal with situations that may arise.

Baby blue is a wonderful color to wear if you do not want to appear a know-it-all, when you are beginning either a relationship, a project (where you are confident about your position, because this will not convey strong authority), or a brainstorming session with friends. For it tells others that you are just starting something and are willing to explore and gather information.

Banana

Vision and reason begin to take on a new twist here, and the bold splendor of yellow finds its exaltation in banana. Wearing banana indicates frankness and teamwork. It is outright honesty that is expected and delivered when you wear banana yellow. For in the true sense, you are out in the open with banana. This is not a color to wear when you are hiding something, for it will be revealed. Wearing yellow tells others that you would never allow yourself to get involved in any "shady" or unscrupulous dealings. Banana is too open an energy to try And wear to fool people, either—honest, up-

front behavior is expected by others and if you are not behaving that way, you will be discovered.

Word of warning here: if you wear too much banana yellow, you may scream "loud-mouth" and others will avoid you at all costs.

Beige (see Oatmeal)

Black

Black is the shade that says, "Take me seriously." Black is actually a blending of all the colors visible to us and as a result it has a strong penetrating quality to it. Powerful black absorbs heat and emanates a warm energy.

Black makes the profound statement of being substantial, so black will cause the message of your color choice to be taken very seriously.

Blood Red

Blood red tells others that you are the driving force. Often it is the power behind the throne.

Wear blood red to let others know that

you are in charge and that you are a source of power. This red gives orders, it doesn't take them.

Blueberry

I was once told that there are no blue foods. I immediately responded by saying, "What about blueberries?" The reply was, "Ahhh, but blueberries are not really blue." I never did find a blue food. And I myself came to the conclusion that blueberry is in fact in the purple family. It is in the color blueberry where we first discover the *truth of faith*.

The gift of blueberry is a new truth, honesty, and honor. Many business suits that are called navy are in fact blueberry. This is a color of deeper truth, something beyond what we see in our daily lives. It's darker than pure navy. Wear blueberry when you are willing to uncover the truth and not afraid to express it.

Blue-Green (see Teal)

Blue-Red (see Magenta)

Blush (see Soft Pink)

Bone (see Ivory)

Brick

Brick is a combination of the earth tones of brown and red. Brown is about family and nature, and the survival energy of red is well served in small doses with brown. Wearing brick tells others that you are a survivor and will do whatever it takes to survive. A large percentage of brick in your home signifies that stability is very important to you.

Bronze (see Brown)

Brown

Brown is the tone of our soil. It is from the earth that our food comes, and so it is the color brown that indicates back to basics, nature, and anything natural or "real." Brown detests pretense and will not tolerate it. The family of brown in general is down-to-earth and real. Wear brown when being who you are is more important than being who others want you to be.

Buff (see Honey)

Burgundy

The large amount of purple lends burgundy its intuitive nature. It is the color that others trust. While burgundy contains the drive of red, it adds the intuition of purple, which leads others to trust your motives.

Wear burgundy when you wish to be deliberate about your ambition but creative enough to trust your own instincts.

The calming elements of purple soften the red and ease the spirit.

Burnt Orange

Burnt orange conveys confidence. It is the color that you wear when you need to give directions to others and have them completely understand what is required of them.

This color has a double edge to it, however. Burnt orange can also lend an air of false confidence and credibility to the wearer.

Since pure orange lends ease to whatever we do, it is in burnt orange that we hide our physical ailments. Burnt orange can help disguise our fear of the truth. But, it is also the color of discrimination, and we may instinc-

tively reach for it when we have determined our personal issues.

Butter

In the softest of yellows we find freedom from irrational feelings. We begin to sort out and think through our feelings. When you wear butter, buried feelings begin to emerge. Butter yellow may isolate us from others, for while it is a soft inviting color, we wear it when we need solitude to sort through our feelings.

Butter also promotes healing of "mental" wounds. You will be drawn to butter when you are in a contemplative mood, and others don't know that, so have patience with them. For your solitude may seem like depression, and others may annoy you by continually asking about your mood.

In butter we reflect our need to commune with ourselves, and this is often uncomfortable to those around us, who are drawn to the jovial nature of yellow.

Camel (see Mocha)

Canary

"Sing like a canary" is the cliché, and it's fairly true! Canary is a bright, effervescent color that will draw others to you like a magnet. People who wear canary are often the talkers in the group. They may not always say the most intelligent things, but what canary lacks in intellect, it makes up for in spunk.

Canary yellow can be associated with gossip, so it may not be the best color to wear to the office. It may not allow others to hold you in the best light. Then why even wear it? Because it does convey organizational skills, for example. Don't rule out wearing canary, just wear it sparingly.

Cantaloupe

A bit of the whimsical and wild begins in cantaloupe. Your delicate touch will be evident when you wear cantaloupe, but all the while conveying that while your tactics may be unconventional, you'll get the task at hand done. Others will trust you and not know why.

Cantaloupe will not agitate, which is good when you have to work closely with people for long periods of time. Like the inspirations of pure orange, cantaloupe inspires you as well as those around you. Like most colors, cantaloupe will tend to effect the wearer first, then others. Since most orange tones are motivational, this can help out quite a bit when we need an extra bit of energy.

Carrot

Carrot can get a project moving! When you wear carrot, it helps make instructions to others clear and less threatening by simply promoting understanding. In this way it assists in putting a stalled project back on track.

Don't overdo the amount of carrot or it can cause others to be unable to concentrate. Carrot naturally inspires, but it can irritate if you wear too much.

Celadon (see Celery)

Celery

Interestingly, this is a color that has become more prominent over the years. A light fun energy, celery supplies the harmony to any situation. Don't expect deep heartfelt discussions, because this is not the place for them.

Where compatibility and harmony are important, celery is best. This color promotes safety for it doesn't pressure others into thinking that "a big talk" is coming. Others can relax and be themselves around celery. A great emotional healing color because of its soothing nature.

Charcoal (see Gray)

Chamois (see Honey)

Chartreuse

Chartreuse boldly announces to others that you have no emotional secrets. In fact, you are so out in the open about them, you may announce them rather loudly. Chartreuse is not worn by those with inhibitions, so it follows that anyone wearing it is up-front and will be truthful with you.

The boisterous energy of chartreuse can unfortunately overshadow the element of an openhearted warmth that is radiated by those who wear it. In truth, everyone wishes they had the loving openness that chartreuse emits.

Cherry

Since red is often thought of as the color of vibrant sexual energy, wear this color when you are ready for the experiences that it will attract into your life.

This is a great color to wear when you are ready to ignite the fire. Cherry is both a happy and a freeing energy which communicates that you are here to either work or defend yourself.

Chocolate Brown (see Brown)

Clear Bright Red (see Red)

Cobalt

Close to electric blue, cobalt is the more regal of the two. Its message of authority is more subtle. It is a more meditative, thinking color. While electric will jump on a dime, cobalt will tell others that you reflect and contemplate the best course of action.

The color of twilight best describes Cobalt. It is the time when we are preparing for the next phase of our day. Cobalt is a wonderful transition color. It tells others that you are flexible and ready to accept the next phase your current project may take on.

Wear cobalt in business if you are confident, not cocky. It will let others know that you are not afraid to dig in and get the work done. Your flexibility is the key here: don't wear cobalt unless you are willing to be flexible, for others will expect it of you.

Cocoa (see Brown)

Coffee *(see Brown)*

Copper *(see Brown)*

Coral

Coral soothes us and allows us to work without much effort. Coral also teaches us with its quiet confidence. When you wear the color coral, it tells others that you are naturally friendly. A very positive color, negative folks may shy away from you when you wear it. Coral emits love and acceptance.

Cornflower *(see Periwinkle)*

Cotton Candy

This is the softest red. So much white has been added that the drop of red only gives it the slightest hint of pink. Cotton candy has a faint warmth to it. There is no commitment here. It tempts with the idea that maybe there is a drop of passion inside. Not a lot. But enough. Wear cotton candy when you need a little energy, but don't want to come on strong.

However, there is not enough communi-cation energy emanating from this color to create ideal group participation. The coolest of reds, it is also the most detached or devoid of feeling.

Cranberry *(see Burgundy)*

Cream *(see Ivory)*

Crimson

Deep red merges red with the absorption of black, and black is the color that takes in all the colors. Wear crimson when you are in a deep place of contemplation. For crimson allows deep sadness to be felt. Wear crimson when you need to retreat and recharge. You can use it to stay inside for as long as you need to.

Dark Tomato Red *(see Blood Red)*

Deep Periwinkle *(see Periwinkle)*

Denim *(see Marine Blue)*

Eggplant

This is the color of true grandiosity. Opulence hides the darkness of eggplant. Things are not as good as they appear with eggplant. If you choose to wear eggplant, you may be stifling your own creativity.

Hiding from one's creativity is indicated here. This is a safe color to wear in a corporate environment as you are telling others that you do not need to be self-expressive to function.

Eggshell (see Ivory)

Electric Blue

Like its name, electric blue is vibrant, intense, and very energetic. It is the choice to stand out. Wear electric blue when you want your presence known. In electric, you are in control of yourself and can handle any difficult situation that may arise. It is the calm of blue mixed with the flair for self-expression that finds itself with electric blue.

This is not the color to wear in a corporate environment. It is too full of self-expression and it may cause a rift with colleagues, for it is by far the most independent of all the blues.

Cobalt and royal are the more calm cousins; they are not as dramatic and can be worn as suits in the proper setting. For this reason, I gave them their own headings.

Emerald

Sparkling and bright, emerald is the perfect color to wear when you are clear and up-front about your motives. The perfect color to wear when you are unafraid to take new emotional risks. Emerald is the color that women reach for when they are ready for a new relationship, for the pure energy of an open heart will attract people to you.

Wear emerald to show love and openness to others. While it creates the energy to begin something new, it also carries with it the powerful follow-through of green. Others will trust you to be steadfast in your ability to complete your tasks. In short, emerald is the symbol of mature love, a love that will not fizzle out, that goes beyond the passion of red, that will endure.

Evergreen

As we get to the deeper side of the green spectrum, we move into the hibernation part of green. Unlike the renewal associated with the green of spring, evergreen is the green of winter and lies dormant, making little change. Evergreen is often married to tradition and is not an experimental color.

Wear evergreen when you wish to appear steady and unchanging. It tells others that you are very attentive to detail and don't mind the seemingly menial tasks that would drive some people crazy. Evergreen is a wonderful completion color.

However, change is hardest for evergreen, which craves consistency. If the need for security is too strong in an individual, it can manifest itself in a desire to control and overpower others.

Don't worry if evergreen is the color you most love to wear! What evergreen lacks in imagination, it makes up for in moral values and reliability. Lurking behind the color of evergreen is the heartfelt sincerity associated with all greens.

Forest Green (see Evergreen)

Fuchsia

Here the razzle-dazzle-hot passion of red stops one step of maturity. Fuchsia says, "I'm here, I have energy, and I'm ready!" It is the spirited and passionate energy of fuchsia that makes it the color to wear to freely express yourself.

The instinctive knowing quality of red stops short in fuchsia. I would not recommend wearing fuchsia for a first meeting, since it enhances playfulness and adds an air of the old-fashioned feminine mystique. It may detract from what you are trying to say. Unless of course, you're an inventor. Fun, unique, silly, clever, impish, anytime spells fuchsia. Wear it to dare.

Geranium

This geranium is an orange/red. Since orange is emotion and movement, and red symbolizes birth, it combines the two well, for geranium is perfect to wear when you are ready to present new ideas.

Keep in mind that since red dominates here, it always represents the movement of the idea, not the conception. This might not be the best color to wear in a room full of people who are brainstorming ideas.

Ginger

When you wear a suit or professional outfit in ginger, it gives the message to others that you can be relied upon to get the job done. Wear ginger when you are willing to complete a task alone, but don't despair, you will soon find others joining in to assist you.

Inspiration is the key to orange, and

others will want to be a part of your productive energy. In certain tribes, ginger is the sacred color of procreation; things will multiply and increase around ginger. It is a wonderful color to wear to win a new account at work.

If you sell anything where profits are expected from you, ginger is a good choice to wear since it promotes trust. Ginger is the perfect color to wear when meeting the boss, since it can also create a belief in your ability to increase capital.

Gold

The regal quality associated with gold is not lost in the wearing of it. Gold conveys the feeling that you treasure yourself and others. The energy of yellow moves away from the more day-to-day intellectual pursuits and enters the realm of the "mind" or spiritual side of thought with gold.

Now, most of us don't realize the far-reaching power or statement that gold can make, but think for a moment of Anne Klein II or Givenchy jewelry. A large part of both faux jewelry manufactures are in gold, and they are large pieces. When you wear some of the collections with the proper gold jewelry, it makes a magnificent impact!

Thinking beyond the mundane day-to-day thoughts is indicated by the wearing of gold, and we leave behind our self-serving be-

havior and begin thinking of others. If you are interested in gaining a promotion at work, for example, gold is a wonderful touch to add to your clothing to make the "powers that be" aware that you are thinking of the good of the whole.

Golden Brown (see Ginger)

Goldenrod (see Canary)

Golden Yellow (see Canary)

Grape

Wear grape when you need to delve into something and make discoveries. Grape is the color of the investigator.

Pride also finds its home in grape. Those who keep their vanity hidden often seek out grape. Wear grape yourself when you do not wish to answer questions. Others will stay away from the aloofness of grape. You are safe from prying questions behind the cloak of grape.

Grapefruit

Yellow itself represents the intellect, and grapefruit is the beginning of the social yellows. It tells others that you are available for interesting conversations.

No deep thought takes place in grapefruit, for wearing it informs others that you are beginning to look outside your own mind for answers. Grapefruit conveys our willingness to listen to another person's point of view.

When we wear grapefruit, others will approach us and tell us the bitter truth. We may not like what we hear, but when we don the color grapefruit we demonstrate our willingness to listen nonetheless.

Gray

Gray says: "I take no sides, I have no opinions." Gray makes a terrific neutral, because when you wear it you let others know that you stand in the middle of the road, and have no answers and make no judgments.

Mix gray tonally (lighter and darker gray), or use a color to lend energy to the "middle of the road" message of gray. One word of warning here: if you do place a color with gray, it's bound to make that color's message stronger.

Gray Blue (see Marine Blue)

Gray Navy (see Marine Blue)

Greige (see Oatmeal)

Honey

An emotional desire to connect is indicated with honey. The need to move closer to things and people that represent love is indicated when one wears honey. Movement toward a gentler feeling is a definite pull here. There is a warmth which emanates from honey that draws softness and love to it.

A wonderful color to wear when a connection is required and you are willing to let it happen.

Hot Pink (see Fuchsia)

Hunter

Straightforward, bold, and strong describe hunter green. Hunter begins the trek into the valley of the hidden. It is not willing to divulge the secrets it has kept in its heart. Insecurity lurks in this dark green.

Hunter green is well matched to the abrasive personality that needs to prove it is "right," when in reality, it is only hiding feelings, burying them in a heart that is perhaps already wounded.

Men tend to wear hunter green to maintain detachment from their feelings while they hunt. If a hunter became emotionally attached to an animal while trying to kill it, he would not succeed in his mission. Such is the power of hunter green. It is very effective at helping us hide how we really feel. The greatest benefit of hunter is it can protect your feelings from others.

Icy Aqua (see Purple)

Icy Blue (see Sky Blue)

Icy Green (see Mint)

Icy Lemon Yellow (see Icy Yellow)

Icy Pink (see Cotton Candy)

Icy Purple (see Purple)

Icy Yellow

A cooling of one's true feeling is indicated by icy yellow. The cheery quality of yellow is made aloof here. A desire to work independently of others begins to emerge.

This is the color that needs to be alone, to think on its own. Icy yellow is about detachment and helps the wearer keep their feelings away from the thinking process. Wear icy yellow when things need to be given careful consideration.

Indigo

For many years I was certain that indigo blue was of the purple family. But indigo actually is right in the middle, and it derives equal energy from both purple and blue. It is the color of intuition.

Indigo combines truth with faith, creating a very powerful combination.

Of all the colors indigo is the most self-assured color. Indigo lets the world know that you know who you are and don't waver. It indicates that you are capable of quick decisions and are certain of your choices. Unlike any other color, it exudes a mature confidence, drawing on an inner sense of knowing that only comes from a spirit that can not be broken.

Ink

The darkest of all blues. Ink is before blackness. It is the color that keeps its truth hidden.

It wishes no one to know its secrets, therefore it never quite reveals who it is. It is a color to wear when you are gathering information but wish to reveal nothing.

While it represents the search for truth, it moves away from communication and into absorption. It gathers, it does not give.

Ivory

Ivory is where a desire to become involved again is just beginning to surface. There is also the idea that taking one step farther in some situation would be wise. The idea behind this is that ivory is perfect to wear when you have been resisting something for a long time, but are ready to begin to move toward it.

Unlike the deflective quality of white, where purity reins, ivory has begun to mature and deepen the need to get involved again.

Wear ivory when you are ready to take a chance. Notice that others wear it when they are about to change their point of view on something that perhaps they've been fixed on for a long time.

Kelly

Kelly is the perfect color to wear to achieve harmony with mind and spirit. That is why city dwellers benefit so greatly from a day in the country!

While we may bury our past hurts in the heart, wearing kelly will bring them to the surface and allow us to face them. Kelly green helps stimulate the heart again.

Kelly reveals that you play your life straight from the heart. There are no hidden meanings to you! When you wear kelly, your message is that you are open and available. It also communicates that you can make decisions swiftly, for you are close to what your heart tells you.

If your spirits are low, kelly will help pick them up. For it is in being attracted to kelly that we know we are finding hope again. It is the color to wear to get back into life again. I've found widows (or anyone who has suffered a loss) will begin to wear kelly when they are rejoining life. Kelly signifies that your heart is once again open to new relationships. Wearing kelly can also tell others that you are feeling the need for love and affection.

Jade (see Emerald)

Lavender

Lavender is not the color for intellectuals. It is a debutante's color, for it loves supporting noble causes. Anything that involves a social gathering is a wonderful place to show up in lavender, for social grace and being a gracious hostess are implied when one wears lavender.

The person wearing lavender will always be the person who is doing something out of love.

The feeling of someone who does nothing but socialize can be the impression left when lavender is worn to a business meeting. You may not be trusted to get the job done if you show up wearing lavender in a professional setting.

Lemon

While canary is bright and light, lemon takes a serious departure. Lemon is being worn more and more by women in the office, and I feel that it is indicative of their ability to speak up and have their intelligence and contribution recognized.

People who wear lemon are not afraid of letting their thoughts be known and will stand up for what they believe. Lemon yellow will get you called upon, and others will expect you to have thought through what you say and be able to back it up. If you wear lemon you tell others that you think things out and are able to defend your position without fear.

This is a wonderful color to wear when you know you are right in a particular situation but cannot bring yourself to speak up yet. Rest assured, however. If you wear lemon, you will be called upon to voice your opinions.

Light Cranberry (see Rose)

Light Orange (see Peach)

Light Purple (see Lilac)

Lilac

When we wear lilac, we carry the reminder to others to gently slow down and enjoy. Lilac is not the color to wear if you want to grind out work. Lilac brings harmony to the workplace when you wish to tell others that you are available to enjoy what you are doing and slowly create something of beauty. Lilac is a wonderful color to wear to a relaxing or joyous occasion, particularly a wedding.

Lime

Lime invites depth of thought and feeling. While only we can decide to undertake the analysis of a heartfelt matter, lime green can generate the feeling of security needed to begin. Lime can inspire others to trust you with their innermost secrets. One note of warning here: do not try to use lime green to falsely gain another's confidence; part of the property of green is that while others may open up to you, it will only happen if your own heart is open and your motives are pure. Lime will not hide your secrets while others reveal theirs; it will act as a catalyst for all involved.

This is why lime green will not be worn by executives. When it comes to strategic planning, lime green is too emotional a color to wear; it would not project a feeling that you are levelheaded enough to handle company responsibility.

Remember that lime delves deep into the heart to uncover hidden truths.

Linen (see Oatmeal)

Magenta

Magenta is the administrator's color. It tells others that you have good organization skills, that you are able to figure things out on your own and don't need a whole lot of prodding. Detail-oriented people often gravitate to magenta. Also, this is a wonderful color to wear when applying for an administrative job in the arts.

Magenta communicates that you are a good friend, for when you wear magenta, you will not forget the little details that make people feel special.

Mahogany (see Burgundy)

Marine Blue

The most interesting thing about blue in the fashion world is that it seems that every year there's a "new" blue (it's usually an "old" blue given a new name). After Operation Desert Storm, the "new" blue the following season was marine blue. Now, while that color has existed for quite some time, suddenly it was being mixed with everything. It was, at the time, being seen as the new navy blue.

The element of true blue is always present, and it softens the seriousness of navy, although in marine it becomes more honest and forthright until we reach the trust status of navy blue.

Mauve

Mauve may be useful when working with people with personality disorders, for it encourages creative problem solving. Kindness, gentleness, and helpfulness are inherent in mauve.

Wear mauve when you do not wish to wallow in your feelings, for while this brings the ability to feel, it does not bathe itself in feelings. When you wear mauve in a work environment, others will perceive you as their gentle and supportive friend. In mauve, we find the combination of gentleness and intuition that is an extremely powerful combination. A delicate sensitivity is the impression that mauve gives out. Mauve is a message to others that you can help guide them.

Medium Purple (see Lavender)

Midnight Blue (see Ink)

Mint

The soft caring of green is found first in mint green. Mint itself is the softest shade of green, and the most calming. Intense pursuits are not on the agenda here! Others will seek out your advice if you wear mint, for you lack the stern judgment that others fear.

If you are seeking to diffuse a tense situation, the loving calm of mint is just the ticket. If you wish to be nonthreatening and set an example of love and acceptance for others, then mint is the color for you as well.

Wearing mint is calming for a potentially volatile situation. However, it is not a color for negotiating!

Mint avoids emotional confrontation, however, and is not a good color to wear if you wish to have a heart-to-heart with someone to express your feelings.

Mocha

Mocha has softened brown's meaning of back-to-basics and nature. The deflective quality of white enters the picture to mix with an air of resistance to it. Not wanting to get too deeply involved in heavy matters is indicated when mocha is worn. There is a need to keep things light, but there is an attachment to the past of some kind. While there is a need to escape the past, there is also a need to stay connected to it.

This is a color that needs to be worn. If there is a connection to mocha, it is necessary to be connected to your angst.

Moss (see Hunter)

Mustard

When you wear mustard it indicates that you are capable of deep thought. It can also denote a strong attachment to family; it can convey that the person wearing it puts family before all else.

If you wear mustard it implies that you are detail-minded. If you are an assistant, it can aid a boss greatly to have you on her team. If you are a boss, it can reassure a nervous client that you will attend to every detail that is of importance to her.

Mustard conveys the feeling that one is unafraid to do hard work.

Navy

Navy says that you are a creative conformist. Wear navy if you tend to be too emotional in your communications with others, for it will detach you and calm you down. This is why navy became a great corporate color. It is a color to wear to a meeting when you want to close the deal. Since navy blue represents truth in the "truest" sense of the word, it is an excellent choice for a first-time business meeting.

When you wear navy blue in a business setting, you tell others that you are committed to honesty and truth. It shows that you are trustworthy and honorable in business. Navy blue creates a calming, authoritative appeal. I find no coincidence in the fact that the majority of airline and other travel-related uniforms are primarily navy blue.

Oatmeal

Hints of being connected to family and deeply rooted issues are beginning to surface with oatmeal. A blending of the need to stay detached and the need to be connected is the pull when one wears this color.

There is no commitment, but there is no leaving either. The inability to make a decision is indicated here. When things are undecided, there is a draw to wear oatmeal.

Off-white (see Ivory)

Olive

Olive goes in and out of fashion as a wardrobe basic depending upon fashion trends. Since olive mixes the pure openness of green with the down-to-earth quality associated with brown, it is often worn as a neutral.

Wearing olive grounds the openhearted attitude of green with the practicality of brown. Why olive instead of brown?

Often brown offers us little personally in the way of energy, while the element of green brings about the ability to stay committed in our hearts. Olive suggests that you are grounded and not apt to make radical changes or do anything that isn't well thought out. It gives the impression that you are not hasty.

What olive lacks in spontaneity, it makes up for in dependability. Others will be drawn to you for your solid approach to things. Wearing olive will give the impression that you are able to handle whatever comes your way.

Like navy, olive remains in the fashion spectrum, while it can be worn as a neutral.

Orange-Red (*see Geranium*)

Orchid (*see Lilac*)

Oyster (*see Ivory*)

Pale Lavender (*see Lavender*)

Pale Lemon Yellow (*see Lemon*)

Pastel Pink (*see Soft Pink*)

Pea

Pea green begins to hide and diffuse the openness of green. If you see someone wearing pea green, they may be hurting inside and trying to heal by reaching outside themselves to feel better. Pea green will elicit attention and caring from others; this may be something that's needed, so it's not necessarily a bad thing.

I once had a client who was wearing a pea green sweater and brown jeans when we first met. I immediately asked her if she was going through a sad time, perhaps losing a relationship or missing her family. She was startled and told me that she and her husband we splitting up and she did in fact miss her mother terribly. In fact, she was planning a trip back to visit her parents in the near future. The brown had indicated her "roots," while the pea green told me that she had mixed feelings about the breakup.

Pea green lets others know that you are

hurting and will draw people to you who wish to be there for you.

Peach

Peach is about service. It is the gentlest of all the oranges, but it is in no way "weak." It is the color that emits joy. Peach is heard in a soft way and helps to clarify confusion. It is a clear color that communicates quite clearly.

It lends a gentle energy to those who wear it, not allowing an energy drain. Others will be attracted to the self-sufficiency of peach. Wear peach to gain a sense of yourself and to learn a new confidence. It is also a color that helps one to feel grounded and serene.

The weakness of peach? It may also convey that you don't see your own worth.

Peacock

This is a most brilliant blue, much like the feathers on a peacock. It is the color that imaginations wear. Peacock means creativity and is often worn by those who find themselves answering to no one.

Wear peacock when you wish to appear humble and not overstate your own message. While this is a wonderful color to wear to your first art gallery opening (if you are the artist or focal point), it is not a good choice to wear to a board meeting where you are in charge, for it can be a humbling color. Peacock has never seen his brilliance. He struts his beauty in front of all, always underestimating what his own worth is—not the color to wear to communicate in the corporate world. Whereas humility for an artist can be perfect.

Peacock is a wonderful power color because it allows you to simply blend in when you don't wish to overshadow others with your brilliance.

Periwinkle

Wear periwinkle when you seek solutions in a peaceful way. Periwinkle will not promote arguments. In fact, you will find that it will have a calming effect on those around you. It states that you are solution oriented *not* winning oriented. It is a perfect color to wear when you are presenting an idea to others who often play "devil's advocate."

Pewter (see Gray)

Pineapple

Pineapple gives the impression that you don't tax yourself with hard work and details. If you are a boss, this is the perfect color to wear if you are speaking to your employees. It transmits that you would never work them too hard, for you yourself wouldn't work to the point of exhaustion. (It is rare to find a workaholic that would wear this color, let alone be attracted to it.) The loose color approach to work is indicated with pineapple.

Pineapple brings you into the present. It is a great vacation color since it immediately helps you unwind and take your mind off pressures elsewhere. In so doing, it can also bring insight into a situation by allowing you to stop focusing on it.

Wearing pineapple will make others seek you out as an escape from their present pressures. They will look to you for a sense of solace and assistance putting things into perspective. You may draw to you people who are wound too tight and need loosening. Don't worry for if you're wearing pineapple, you're already there.

Pine Green (see Evergreen)

Plum

The giving of oneself is indicated with plum. However, there is a neediness that hides in plum that can scare others away. No one likes to feel like someone will cling to them or be a burden. Plum can take humility to the breaking point.

Poppy (see Geranium)

Powder Blue (see Baby Blue)

Powder Pink

Powder pink is a very unobtrusive color; wear it when you want to be present and accounted for, but not center stage. This is precisely why this color is chosen for bridesmaids' dresses.

Pumpkin

Pumpkin inspires the following of rules, evoking a sense of serenity and sincerity. We'll follow a person wearing inspirational, gentle pumpkin before condemning them.

Pumpkin also inspires edifying talks with others. You may even receive credit for having thought or said something brilliant that you didn't say.

Wearing pumpkin may attract people that are good for us as well, those interested in our well-being. Pumpkin makes intentions clear. Pumpkin worn in close quarters can be very effective. However, as an authoritative color it can alienate or irritate. Therefore, pumpkin may be perfect to wear in preparing a speech; but wearing it to give a speech may alienate a large group of people.

Wear pumpkin when you know what needs to get done. Completing something without an exact goal in mind may not be possible, for pumpkin lacks focus.

Purple

Purple takes us out of "comprehension" and into higher knowledge, which is where faith resides. Since the color purple receives its energy in the form of visions and images, it often relies upon the intangible as fact. A "fact" that would drive any analytical person crazy.

Purple is never in a hurry. Selfish interests vanish as the thoughts turn to those of "greater" good. The purple spectrum is a gentle push in the direction of trusting true spiritual beliefs. Purple can be regal or shy, and it makes us more sensitive to ourselves and others.

Faith is the main thrust of purple. While other colors may lend the impression that we are capable *people,* purple tells others that we have capable *imaginations.*

Orchid is the flower most often chosen for easter—the resurrection. High priests wear purple robes on high holy days as well. Purple is also the most spiritual of the colors, for it aligns itself with powers not seen by the eye.

Putty (*see Oatmeal*)

Raspberry

Raspberry combines the purple of higher consciousness with the willfulness of red. The passionate determination of raspberry wants you to get the message and integrate it right away.

Wear raspberry when you are confident in your decisions and are ready to receive nothing but support from others. The message of raspberry is: "I know what I'm doing, follow me."

Rich Cranberry (*see Burgundy*)

Rose

Rose finds itself with the softened meaning of red. Rose is a cooling of the passion that gets a project going, but what it lacks in initiative, it makes up for in the organizing area.

There is also a natural detachment from the need to make something happen that is implied here.

There is really nothing at stake in getting something going. So follow-through is easier. Rose also draws attention to the wearer as a warm person.

Rose-Brown (see Brick)

Royal

Confident is the key word here. The independent flair of royal blue comes on strong. Where electric may jump in and cobalt may wait and see, it is in royal that confidence is found.

It is not the color to wear to a powerful meeting, however, since its strength lies in its individuality and not in the ability to be a team player. Royal is a wonderful confidence builder. It gives the impression that you are self-assured and calm.

Ruby

Ruby red is connected to sexual urges, the calling of nature, being in touch with your own "gut" instincts. Ruby's brown tone is connected to the earth, which gives the message of family and values. Although red is a self-motivating energy, the brown mixes with it to give support to the idea of serving others. Wear ruby when you are in the space to serve and help others.

Remember Dorothy's ruby slippers in *The Wizard of Oz?* Ruby contains a sparkle of joy, the passion of red, and is well placed here.

Rust

Rust signifies the completion of the idea phase. It is the time to dig in and prepare for the task at hand. Wear rust to inspire yourself and others to undertake a lengthy task that requires concentrated effort. Rust is not the color to wear for great inspiration, for it promotes concentration.

Wearing rust tells others that you are not interested in being a leader, you are quite content to be the follow-through person.

Watch for buried anger from someone wearing all rust. If you are questioning someone's motives and they are wearing rust, trust your instincts.

Sage (see Olive)

Salmon

The expansion of consciousness and awareness of brotherhood begin in salmon. The color of magnificent sunsets brings with it humanity and equality. In salmon, others will begin to see your worth and reflect it back to you.

The inspiration from salmon comes in the form of example, creating the understanding that it is with faith we find our inspiration. For in salmon we find the energy of divine justice. The only inspiration available to us is through an inner belief that what we're doing is "right."

Wear salmon when you believe in your convictions and others will follow you. Salmon draws others to you, because they want to learn how they can have what you have.

Scarlet (*see Crimson*)

Shocking Pink (*see Fuchsia*)

Silver

The glow of silver brings to life the cool quality of metal. It brings forth a cool detachment, implying that you are well put together and collected. Silver suggests wealth in an understated way.

Silver adds a cool confidence to any combination. Whatever combination you wear, with silver it means cool confidence.

Sky Blue

Expansion. The idea that there is something beyond what we currently can see, touch, and feel. When you wear sky blue, you tell others that the truth sets you apart for you are unique. You are a thinker and solve problems creatively. Sky blue is an excellent color to wear when you are in need of defusing a potentially difficult situation.

Soft Fuchsia (*see Rose*)

Soft Pink

Soft pink is a light flirtatious color that likes to be desired, rather than to desire. The term *coquette* is well placed with the flirtatious soft pink, for it is receptive. Soft pink summons assistance. It's the color to wear if you want others to help you. Don't wear it if you want to prove you're a team leader, no one will believe you.

Soft Purple (see Purple)

Soft Rust (see Rust)

Stone (see Gray)

Sunset

Sunset is a different blending of fire red with the movement-oriented orange. This color takes action even if we don't. If you wish something to happen, wear sunset and it will propel you into action. Sunset will also tell others that you are headed in the direction of your goals.

Tan (see Beige)

Tangerine

In tangerine, orange sheds its inhibitions and helps lift our repressed feelings through action.

Fun is the key to tangerine; it is a sociable, party color. Wearing tangerine tells others that you'll always find the good in them, thus making you a requested guest.

Tangerine implies slimness because it is so active, inspiring physical activity.

Superficiality may also be present in tangerine—in order to find acceptance, one may wear tangerine when their motives are less than honorable. However, because of the nature of tangerine, others can see through the charade.

Taupe (see also Oatmeal)

Teal

Teal is very close to aqua, but there are a few subtle differences that are worth noting. Teal combines green first, then blue. Since green dominates, teal is the color of close friendship.

Wearing teal in a new social setting is a fabulous choice! You will be perceived as a very caring, honest friend to have. Teal is also a wonderful color to wear to promote trust from the opposite sex.

Terra-cotta (see Rust)

True Red (see Red)

Turquoise

This mixture of communicative blue with abundant green tells others that you are strong and not afraid to ask for, and receive, what you want. Turquoise has a silent strength. When wearing turquoise one expresses a willingness to work and be responsible for her actions.

While it may seem to be a frivolous color, it is really a very earnest color. When you wear turquoise you make a quiet statement of capability and gentleness. You tell others that while you may *seem* soft and very pliant, you are able to handle yourself in any situation.

Turquoise is not very flexible—however, it gives out a very strong message of security. Others will feel they can depend upon you to be there for them. There's no hidden agenda to turquoise.

Vibrant Aqua (*see Aqua*)

Watermelon

The spirited warmth of watermelon says energy! A perfect color to add to your casual wardrobe, it adds the surprise element of self-motivated energy.

Watermelon comes into vogue every few years as the new hot color and you'll find everyone wearing it. Since it lacks the seriousness of the deeper reds, it is best worn outside the workplace.

Wheat (*see Honey*)

White

Unlike black, which absorbs all the colors, white deflects all the colors. The image of cleanliness is true, however white does not get involved in anything either. Therefore, while white is seen as clean and pure, it is also alone and isolated. It does not touch or truly get involved. So, choose the white you wear with care.

Wine

A person who wears wine may secretly desire to conform but wants others to think they are different.

Wine may make one appear to be inconsistent and indecisive if they wear too much of it. Wine tells others that while you are a passionate being, you also rely upon inspiration and have thoughts of your own.

What a wonderful color to close out the 1970s! A decade where that was the struggle for women everywhere. While very few of us wish to return to that era, some women still wear wine, for it reminds them of a time when they stood up for what they believed in.

Yellow Green (see Chartreuse)

Chapter Fifteen

MIXING YOUR METAPHORS – WHAT HAPPENS WHEN YOU MIX COLORS?

The truth is that how you mix colors is a part of personalizing your style and making your message congruent.

> **Tip:** Always mix patterns with the same tonal intensity.

When you add a scarf to an outfit, make sure that the tone, shade, or hue has the same intensity as the outfit. In other words, only mix shades with shades, hues with hues, understand? I know it seems simple, but many women will put a dark blue scarf with a light green outfit and say, "but blue and green match . . . don't they?"

If you're mixing a few solid colors, you can tie the look together with a scarf, *but* make sure that the tonal intensity is the same. If you're using all bright colors, adding a pastel scarf that has all the same colors won't work. But, when you add a scarf that has the same tonal intensity, it works. That is perfect tonal mixing.

PATTERN MIXING

This area is by far the trickiest to understand. I've seen fashion experts who mess this up. (Since I work with them, I generally don't tell them.) The rules don't change here either. When it comes to mixing patterns, the key is . . . match tonal intensity! I don't mean to beat you over the head with it, but repetition is the mother of skill, and it is my goal to make you as skilled as possible.

One final word about coordinating your colors. When designers put together "tonal outfits," it can be marvelous. For example, wearing two blues—say, a navy pant and a sky blue blouse with crisp silver accessories—can look wonderful. While this outfit looks fantastic with jewelry, you can add a scarf, instead. Find a scarf that has the colors you are mixing (red with pink, purple with lavender, etc.), and chances are it will work in with other pieces you already own.

While Dramatics and Trendys can and do get away with quite a bit, just remember not to overcrowd your look. You wouldn't tell someone everything about you the first time you meet them, so don't wear everything you own with one outfit. Less is more (for Sporty, Romantic, Traditional, and Classic)

Obviously, wearing a red dress or a navy suit makes a direct statement, and certain silhouettes *can* be passed among style types. Make sure that any shape with a pattern is *in* your style type, since it's harder to pass off a pattern borrowed from another style type. Obviously, a sundress with a small floral print in a classic silhouette would be avoided by Ms. Romantic, but be conscious of the silhouette you choose.

WEARING COLORS

When someone is wearing solid colors, it is the color closest to eye level that is the color with the dominant message. The colors farther away from eye level fall into a secondary category.

For example, let's say you are wearing a green sweater set and a black skirt. The first impression is that today, matters of the heart are primary to you (this gets more specific if we choose a particular green, but for now let's stay generic). Then, because you are wearing black, I can make a quick assessment that you are serious about whatever emotional state you are in. The darker the green, the more buried your feelings; while the lighter, the more open. If you wear a color with a neutral, the *color* always dominates and the neutral only strengthens the message.

Noticing how people combine colors is a large part of interpreting. Like astrology, the more you know, the more accurate you can be. Now that you have the general meaning of the colors from your style chapter, you can begin to get more specific here.

Before we move on, let me share one final thought here. Don't ever forget about the colors the other person is wearing in business. If you are a salesperson and are hoping to sell a product to a person who is a Traditional and you've never seen her wear red, it may not be wise to wear red to a meeting. However, if your prospect is a Trendy and she wears lots of flamboyant colors, then if *you* wear a navy suit, you may find yourself out the door without the order.

I'm not saying that you should copy them, but within your own style, wearing the right colors can create an instant rapport. While the wrong ones, well, let's just say you may not get the job. Whatever you do, you must do it within your own style.

ACCENT COLORS

Let's move on to accent colors. There are times when a hanky in a jacket pocket can say more to me than a whole outfit. An accent color can be very powerful.

Anything you accessorize with can be an accent color if the piece draws attention to itself. I once worked with a Trendy woman who had a reputation for being very volatile. The day we met she was wearing a brown suede outfit and a pair of yellow earrings that resembled a mobile. Her colors told me that she was feeling very down-to-earth that day, and her choice of accent color clued me into the fact that she was feeling cooperative. Whew!

Had she been wearing red earrings instead of yellow, I would have known that her focus that day was on herself and not on cooperating with others. I therefore would have adjusted my approach to her accordingly; she was after all, the client.

Keep in mind that interpreting is tricky. While green in general pertains to "matters of the heart," there are several subtle ways it can go. That is why in the individual style chapters I give you an overview of each color, in general.

Now comes the question that is most frequently asked: "How come we don't all look alike if many of us wear similar outfits?" Answer: style. Your personal style has a great deal to do with the way you accent an outfit; therefore, the color affects your total look accordingly. A Trendy and a Romantic wearing the same outfit would accent it differently.

As you combine colors, you'll begin to notice which aspect of the color's energy is lending itself to your look. Remember: An accent color directs the way a primary color's energy will be used.

SECTION III

PUTTING IT ALL TOGETHER

Chapter Sixteen

ACCESSORIES – HOW TO WEAR THEM

I've always used accessories to make people notice what I wanted them to.

As a petite woman, I've never wanted people's focus to be down at my feet, that's why shoes are rarely an *accent* for me; however they're important, so let's start there.

SHOES

In 1993 we saw the return of the "platform" shoe. Many of my clients were saying to me, "Never again! I'll never again wear that." Before they could say, "Style," I had them in a pair of mules. It became a good basic spring/summer shoe. It is important, each season, to take stock of your shoes and update them if you need to.

Years ago, I heard that the number-one-selling color was black, except during the summer, when white was the most frequently purchased color.

When it comes to shoes, it is much more important to choose shoes based upon your style than what's "in." When you took the style quiz, you discovered your personal style type. Let's now begin to put it all together by looking at the importance of that choice for you.

Tip: Buy shoes later in the day when your feet have swollen a little. This way your shoes will fit well.

Tip: Huge decorations on shoes shorten the leg. If you are looking to lengthen your legs, buy a plain pump and pass on the buckles and bows.

The **Sporty** woman will have colors that please her in her closet. If she favors hot pink, then her sneakers will reflect that. She is the trendsetter with athletic wear, so she may well have some very trendy types of styles in her closet to go with her sporty outfits.

In general, matching a shoe to your outfit adds to the congruence of your statement. Keep in mind, however, that wearing a patterned dress that has some lime green in it does not necessarily mean you should match shoes to it. When you are trying to find which color from a pattern to accent with, pick the same one for your earrings and shoes.

Tip: if you are either petite or short waisted, when you wear a belt and match it to a shoe, that's fine, but you must match the same color in an earring or scarf to pull the color up and balance yourself.

A **Romantic** woman will have very strappy tie-up silhouettes in almost any color in her closet. She is most comfortable in boots in the winter, as they lend themselves well to the flowing fabrics she enjoys wearing. However, one of my close friends is in the film business and she was the first to rejoice when clogs came back. She even bought herself a pair of mules before I suggested it.

While the color will most likely be black, she may surprise you with a wild-colored boot. In addition, she may buy anything with a floral pattern or with stripes. Her shoes are often fabrics and in colors that reflect an emotion for her.

The **Traditional** woman would never wear ruby red shoes with a ruby red dress. Blue with blue? If it's navy or a Dyeables shoe worn to a wedding, sure. The Traditional woman will take care of her shoes and keep them for years. Open her closet and you'll find lots of neutrals—navy, white, black, taupe, perhaps a red, gray, or one pastel. Very rarely will you find patterned shoes in here.

The **Classic** woman will match shoes to her outfits, but special attention is paid to always be stylish and not too way out. Classic may have some floral-patterned shoes and shoes in a variety of colors. Ms. Classic is not afraid to make a statement with her clothes, but she'd never want others to say, "What's that shoe she's wearing?"

So, in general, a Classic woman may wear a "wow" shoe, but it's always something that looks polished. In her closet you'll find shoes in colors that work with her style of clothing.

A **Dramatic** woman often makes her statement in color, and it doesn't stop at her shoes. She is the first to buy a pair of electric blue shoes or ruby red shoes to match an outfit. This statement is very dramatic in itself and makes her message all the more powerful.

In her shoe closet you'll find at least one shoe from another decade, and she loves sexy shoes!

A **Trendy** woman is the first to buy a style of shoe in what seems to be the most useless silhouette and color, then proceeds to wear it with everything—and wear it well. I have a Trendy friend who bought a pair of red sneakers years ago, and I was aghast! She then wore those sneakers together with everything she owned, from skirts to pants, and they became her calling card for a while. When others started wearing them, she moved on. With a Trendy and shoes, it's "expect the unexpected." If it's "in," it'll be "out" of her closet. Oh, what about my example of electric blue shoes or a ruby red dress? She wouldn't wear either of them, now. Why? Because I'm using them as examples.

PANTY HOSE

When you match a color of hose to a shoe and skirt (or pant), make *sure* they match. Also with a red dress and red shoes, red hose is quite a dramatic or trendy style. While navy shoes, hose, and suit are very traditional.

As a Classic, I typically match my shoes, hose, and skirt. It's easier for me that way. However, every season a new color of hose is introduced (as the shade or hue of the season), and if you want to keep up-to-date, ask in the hosiery department at any major department store. They are quite knowledgeable about the "current" color. If you know what color you like, buying by catalog is another option.

BELTS

Keep an eye on belts every season, they change very fast. Trends often happen by accident: an outfit needs a belt and the stylist on a magazine shoot can only find one—and the photographer is wearing it. It's too big, it gets tied, and the next thing we know, it becomes the belt of the season. (It doesn't always happen like this, but it has.)

When we're going into the holiday season, we know that we're going to see more chain belts, velvet, and beading. However, when we start to see a style out of its "season," then it's probably a trend. As an example, a few years ago velvet belts appeared on the fashion runways early in fall. Since they normally appear for holiday, it was a fad.

SCARVES

As I said previously, a scarf must match tonally to make sense. Here's an example: suppose you are wearing a hunter green dress. You have on a brown belt and matching brown shoes. You choose a scarf with lots of brown in it, but the green is much more kelly than hunter. Does it work?

No. For two different reasons. First, the scarf must match tonally with both the color of the dress and the belt, otherwise you don't match. Second is the fact that by wearing a different green in this case, you are not being congruent with your message. In this case, the brown accent color would become more important than your primary color. Also, interestingly, it tells quite a bit about you. For example, if you mix up your greens like this, you will be conveying emotional confusion, and that can lead people to distrust you and not know why.

So matching your scarf colors is vital if you want others to get a consistent message from you.

By the way, Traditionals are big scarf people. They are the ones who always know how to tie them. Unlike the Sporty bandanna, scarves are Traditional's thing!

JEWELRY

When it comes to jewelry, I could spend hours talking. But I'll break it down simply. There's gold, silver, and colors.

The important thing to remember is that gold is meant to be worn with warm tones: red, orange, or yellow, for example. Green is the dividing line and can go cool or warm easily.

Silver is meant to be worn with the cooler colors. Beginning with green as the divider we then go to blue, which is the natural home of silver, and then on to indigo and purple.

What about navy blue? Is it better with silver or gold? While Navy is a cool tone, it is also considered a neutral, and as such either silver or gold is acceptable here. In addition, any of the neutrals (black, gray, white, brown) can be worn with either gold or silver. Except for brown, which is too warm a tone to mix with silver (although some have done it quite successfully because it does break a rule). In recent years, gray has begun to be worn with gold, but typically that too was a cool tone and only worn with silver.

WATCHES

Personally, I love watches and have quite a few. (Remember, though, I'm a Classic) Silver, gold, and various colors. They're great staples for a business wardrobe. It's amazing how easily a watch adds polish to a look.

What about colors? The whole idea behind colorful jewelry is to add to the outfit, not detract. I'm not going to tell you how much you need to wear, all I'll say is: Less colors, stronger message.

You find a jungle-print dress you *have* to have. It's a green (olive) leaf background with brown, red, orange, and yellow running through it.

You are in love with the red belt it came with. Fine. Red earrings will make it a daytime dress, or find an olive belt with a gold buckle that matches the dress and wear gold earrings.

For petites and fuller sizes, it's a must to match earrings to your belt. For those who are taller, you don't have to match your earrings to your belt, just make sure that the belt doesn't detract from your overall look. Sometimes the belt that comes with a dress cheapens it. Manufacturers don't know everything. The same dress is designed for a lot of different women, so if you don't like the belt, find one that is better suited for you.

A colorful accessory will make it a dress to wear for daytime, while a sophisticated gold or silver watch will make it a dress to wear to dinner.

Make sure that the accessories you choose are appropriate for the time of day and place. If you work for a conservative company, silver or gold only. Colors are fine, but they should blend in, not stick out.

I went to a new dental hygienist recently, and she was wearing red parrot earrings with her dress. The hygienist was a Traditional trying to look Trendy. Oops. A wonderful pair of cloisonné earrings would have been perfect for her. Alas, parrots or fish or any kind of casual earring is best left for the weekend. Watch not only the style you choose, but color.

Make sure your color choice doesn't overpower the outfit, unless you're a Trendy—then do whatever you feel. My rule is that if you're trying too hard to get something to work, it probably doesn't. The fewer colors, the more powerful your statement and the more congruent you appear.

Oh, gosh, I almost forgot pearls! The pearl necklace or earring comes on strong for Traditionals, Classics, Romantics and sometimes Sportys. Remember though, different styles will wear different designs. (Imagine Mariel Hemingway in pearls—she's a true Sporty. While she can wear them and look beautiful, they don't quite fit her natural style.) Dramatics and Trendys will almost never wear pearls, unless to a funeral or a wedding.

Tip: Do watch trends where pearls are concerned. When Barbara Bush was first lady, her three-strand choker was the way to wear a pearl necklace. When Hillary Clinton became first lady, pearl strands dropped, became longer and a much more relaxed look came into vogue. Interestingly, although both Barbara Bush and Hillary Clinton are Traditionals, fashion began to change. This is because as the generations change, the idea of Traditional (or any other style type) gets updated.

BAGS

The old cliché of belts and bags is still true. Match them.

What about Dramatic? Expect a matching bag that makes a statement. Dramatics use fewer colors overall, which makes a greater impact for them. She'll either have a bag for just about every outfit, or a few stop-traffic bags that go with everything.

I have a close buddy who is a Pediatrician and a Trendy. One day, she met me carrying a children's lunchbox, and it wasn't for one of her patients; she was using it as a purse! And it worked! The kids at the hospital had drawn all over her white sneakers, so they matched her "purse." She looked pretty funky, but it suited her!

I'm a former New Yorker, so I never want to attract too much attention to my handbag, but I have a Traditional friend in Dallas who won't go out if her bag doesn't complement what she has on. I'm convinced that she owns a Coach handbag in every color.

Classics tend to have a wide variety of purse styles, so at first glance it may seem that they are scattered in what they buy. For instance, a Classic may have and wear a leather knapsack, which is weekend wear for her. The knapsack style is typically Sporty, but a Sporty considers her leather knapsack dressy, and she'll wear it with a suit. It's how you wear an accessory that makes it a particular style, not necessarily the accessory itself. Sportys have bags that can haul their things, but always in a fabric that works in with their wardrobe.

Romantics usually have woven or cloth bags, although for dressier or work-related occasions they sometimes have leather attachés—although the rule here is loose and unconstructed.

Should you match your bag? This is entirely up to you. Just make sure it's your style!

HATS AND GLOVES

While both hats and gloves in general should match, that's not always the case. Once reserved only for weddings, Trendys and Romantics have changed all that!

Romantics will wear feminine hats that blend with their outfits, then add long dangle earrings and look marvelous. Lace gloves are a perfect choice for her, while a Traditional woman will wear gloves to church, on holidays, or to special gatherings. Delicate lace gloves will complement her pearl earrings and necklaces. She may own a hat or two, but they are always understated, never something glaring.

A Classic woman may have hats that are on the dramatic side—if she wears them. The key to a Classic woman is that no matter what she is wearing, it will be put together in a classic way and that may include a hat or pair of gloves that is the perfect complement to her outfit.

Dramatics have a way of wearing a pair of colorful gloves with a coat and looking fantastic—are you getting the idea that there are few firm rules in fashion? There are rules, the only problem is, they don't apply to everyone. That's why within your own style, you must decide if it works for you.

Trendys will wear the wildest, strangest hats and look absolutely fabulous. Expect weightlifting gloves worn as an accessory where Trendy is concerned!

ACCESSORY TIPS

- Larger earrings take off about five pounds visually.
- For fuller figures and petites, try to match your belts to something up high on your body, like earrings or a hat or scarf, for example. It gives you a longer line and makes you appear more evenly proportioned.
- If you're short waisted, wear a pin on your shoulder rather than the lapel of a jacket. It cuts the visual distance between your ear and where a taller woman would normally place the pin, this creates a visual sense of proportion. Great for petites.
- Always buy your accessories when you buy the outfit. Don't later get caught trying to match a scarf to an outfit hanging at home in your closet!
- If you're a petite, you can measure a print or pattern by your hand size. Hold your hand up to that print, and if it's your hand size or smaller, it's the right size for you.
- Buy your favorite accessory when it's the newest trend; you'll find more of a selection that way.

> **Tip:** For petites—if you have a print you love to wear but discover that it's too large for you, I suggest you take the smallest portion of the pattern and match that color to the accessories. This will minimize the print.

Before we finish accessorizing, here are a few tips on accenting with color. You can use up to two different colors to accent and still keep your statement congruent. After that, when you start mixing too many colors, you'll begin to dilute the impact. So, the most powerful way to use color is:

1. Never accent with more than two colors (in addition to your primary color).
2. Remember that the color closest to eye level will be the most important, *even* if it's the accent color.
3. Color impact is from eye level down. Keep this in mind especially if your boss (or client) is taller than you—a hair accessory may be the dominant color to them.

BUSINESS WARDROBE

Here are a few tips for building a business wardrobe:

1. Read the definition of the colors that appeal to you in the color glossary. For presentations, always wear the color that is most congruent with what you are trying to convey. For example, if you are trying to convey that you are honest, work blue into your wardrobe.

2. Build your work outfits around your three personal colors. This will assure you that you are at the most ease with yourself and your coworkers.

3. Most working women own quite a bit of black. That's fine. Accent your black wardrobe with as many of your three colors as you can.

4. Don't automatically buy a black winter coat. You may find one in another color that is perfect for you. I once worked with a Sporty client who insisted upon buying a long leather coat in a royal blue. This coat looked great on her! It worked with all her looks, and the color was perfect, too. She wore multicolored mittens and scarf with it, and while I thought she looked like a Popsicle, it was her style, and it did look wonderful on her. Consider that your winter coat should suit your personality as well as your style.

SPECIAL OCCASION DRESSING

What's really appropriate for you? Let's do a quick overview of what's expected at each of the gatherings you're invited to.

1. White tie is extremely formal. This is ball gowns only. The invitation will generally say white tie. This needs to be planned as far in advance as possible. For an event of this magnitude, you should definitely work with a personal shopper or have something made.

2. Black Tie is formal. The single largest mistake many women make is wearing a simple knee-length silk dress to a black tie event. Don't allow a cocktail dress to do the job of a formal outfit. Black tie is not semiformal. Avoid the day-to-evening work mistake: *no* suits with pearls! This category needs a dressy dress, a short sequined or chiffon shift would be fine. This is a feminine look. Go through catalogs and magazines. Find pictures that you think are correct for black tie and that appeal to you. Don't rule out an appropriate outfit just because the accessories pictured are not you, that can be changed.

Give yourself at least a month prior to your event to find the right dress. Consider buying this in one of your three personal colors. If you can only find it in black, and want it in a color, you may have to have it made for you by a dressmaker. This is something you can wear a few times a year if it's seasonless. Plan on getting (at the most) five years of wear out of it. If it's in a fabric that is transseasonal or wearable anywhere, it may stretch farther.

Always buy this for the city in which you live. If you live in New York but your sales meeting is in Florida, don't buy for Florida. Remember that the people who you are going to see at the meeting expect you to look like New York. Do stay flexible here, though. If you're attending a wedding in Dallas, darker colors will draw a few stares. Think of the region you'll be visiting.

3. Black Tie Optional—I hate these invitations because they're misleading. This kind of event is trying to say, "Come as you are, but formally."

No, it's not really okay to wear a business suit, or even your silk cocktail dress. But, alas, women do. Remember, this is still a formal event. An elegant pair of pants with a beautiful belt would suffice if pants are in. I believe it's always better to overdress than underdress, but then I'm a Classic.

Consider your style and use your own judgment.

Tip: Consider the hostess's style. Is she a Sporty? Or a Dramatic? That should give you some clue as to what she'll expect of her guests.

---

4. Cocktail Reception—yes, that silk dress is fine here, and knee-length is accept-

able. You can even get away with elegant cotton knits here.

If you choose one of your three personal colors in your wardrobe for any of your special occasions, your accessorizing will be a breeze because you will already own the matching basics: shoes, hose, and accessories.

Remember, don't abandon your style, no matter what the occasion.

Chapter Seventeen

WHAT YOU SHOULD KNOW BEFORE YOU SAY, "CHARGE IT"

TRENDS AND FADS

Years ago, trends came in for a season or two and then were gone. Today, a "trend" is something that you can see beginning one season and over a period of many seasons becomes a wardrobe staple for you. Designers are giving us styles that are wearable for more seasons than ever before.

A fad is something that comes in one season, doesn't last, and is soon gone. Often it's simply a new look that didn't catch on.

Back in 1990, quilting on jackets and patchwork detailing came into style. This was a fad and didn't last.

The way to tell if a style is a trend is to ask yourself if this was around last season. If a "look" picks up steam as the seasons roll along, it's a trend and *not* a fad. In short, a fad comes and goes very quickly, while trends come in and stay for a while.

WHY SOME THINGS BECOME A TREND AND OTHERS DON'T

Streetwear is the look that began with bicycle messengers. The uniform of a professional messenger was lycra bike shorts and a tank top. The trend was called streetwear because, quite literally, the trend began in the "streets."

When bike shorts first appeared, many of us said, "That'll never last. It'll be gone next season." What happened instead was that the fitness craze of the late 1980s coincided with it, and—Whammo! We were soon wearing bike shorts under fancy sweaters!

The bike short soon grew into leggings, and suddenly we were all wearing T-shirts over our shorts and leggings. Then we added blazers. When crochet came in, it went over leggings, and all of this built on the streetwear trend. The return of the palazzo pant was the first move away from this look. Why?

My guess is the new political administration in the White House in 1992.

HOW TO DISCOVER WHAT WE ARE FOCUSING ON NOW

Karl Lagerfeld redefined "Classic" by showing denim being worn with suits. During that season, I remember finding quite a bit of resistance to this new "style."

Right after Desert Storm, denim was back in focus because it was considered a very "American" fabric. The "American" look brought Calvin Klein back into the limelight and made Donna Karan hotter than ever. And suddenly Lagerfeld's brilliant collections from the previous season made perfect sense.

Fashion always takes its cues from national and world affairs. If these events are "big" enough, a fad can easily become a trend. For example, a few years back animal rights activists became a powerful group. Remember the vote in Colorado to outlaw the wearing of fur coats? The following fall season animal-print everything was in! The catch? It had to be *fake*. This inspired a huge trend that by the spring of 1993 became a fad that was called urban safari.

The best way to follow trends is to read the magazines. The majors give you the scoop on what's happening: *Allure, Elle, Essence, Glamour, Harper's, Mademoiselle, Mirabella,* and *Vogue* are the leaders in fashion editorial. They will give you a feel for the new fashions each month.

The big fashion issues to pick up are the spring and fall issues. If you are looking in what I call the "targeted" magazines, remember that the fashions here are directed toward their readers. Ladies Home Journal, Lear's, Redbook, and Woman's Day are a few examples of magazines directed toward a more specific audience and therefore their fashion coverage will be more tailored to their readers and may not reflect all the *trends or fads.*

Each of these magazines is very thorough, but I always recommend reading more than one to get a clear overview of the market.

HOW YOU CAN STAY ON TOP OF THE NEWEST TRENDS AND FORGET THE FADS

Remember when I suggested that you tear pages out of magazines for your collage? I do this every season to update my wardrobe. In general, I find between one and four key items I need to update. If red is the craze this season, I go to my closet. How is my red supply? Can my red Kaspar suit go one more season? Probably (remember I'm a Classic). If the trend is red, you'll find something you love from your favorite designer because everyone will be doing red.

Always buy the "in" color when it's "in" if it's one of your colors. That's the time to replace or add to your wardrobe. Since I've already mentioned designers, let's talk about their style.

DOES THEIR "STYLE" FIT YOURS?

Liz Claiborne became a legend when she began making clothes that fit our *life-style.* She began with missy and blew open the petite industry in the early 1980s. By the end of the 1980s she gave dignity to the full-sized woman with the introduction of her Elizabeth line.

What made Liz Claiborne so successful? Quite simply, her designs can be worn by almost any style type. There isn't a woman I know who can't wear something from one of her many lines. The more popular a clothing line, the more universal their appeal to all the style types.

Often I hear a woman say, "Oh, I'd never wear that manufacturer's clothes." She has an idea of what that vendor's image is, and she doesn't feel it suits her. Yes?

When I say Calvin Klein, your first image is Sporty. But then we think, Traditional and Romantic can work, too. Trendy? Probably some things. Classic? Yes, especially some of his more "classic" looks. Dramatic? Sure.

Don't rule out a designer or label if *once* they didn't work for you. Times change, and designers create new collections all the time.

The same is true of all the popular designers. If someone is "big," chances are they've managed to appeal to quite a few different style types.

Chapter Eighteen

TRAVELING IN STYLE

On my last business trip, I was on the road for ten days and carried one medium-sized suitcase. When I went to the islands last year, I carried a smaller bag and didn't need a thing that I didn't have. I believe that packing, like dressing, is a skill that just takes practice. However, the average person doesn't travel more than once or twice a year, so how could they expect to know what they'll need?

First consider where you are going. For how many days? What can you wash out by hand? Do avoid packing anything that requires dry-cleaning.

Also consider what you'll buy there. If it's a beach community, budget in that you may want to buy a new suit or towel for a souvenir. Buy useful souvenirs. I buy key chains and colorful towels when I go to the Caribbean. All my towels are from places I travel. I have a friend who has a coffee mug collection from everywhere she's been. When she has company, she serves coffee with her travel mugs. It makes for great conversation. And this saves you the trouble of throwing away all those meaningless souvenirs later on.

Before you pack, consider the following:

1. Be familiar with the place you are traveling to. If traveling out of the country, make sure you have any personal medical supplies with you.
2. Bring a waterproof suitcase. I've seen clothes soaked through and ruined by a rainstorm.
3. Try not to travel with luggage that you can't manage; porters are scarce in airports these days.

4. Lugging luggage around can be painful. Invest in a set of wheels to tote your luggage and save your back! Or buy a Travel-pro-type of luggage to carry on the airplane.

A FEW PACKING TIPS

1. Keep a prepacked travel kit ready to go.
2. Use plastic bags to wrap your clothing, since it cuts down on wrinkles. The trick is the trapped air in the plastic!
3. The plastic bag that you roll your shoes in can be reused for dirty laundry.
4. Roll everything to prevent wrinkles. Stuff socks in your shoes.
5. Put shoes and heavier items at the bottom.
6. Always put crushable things, like silk blouses, on top.
7. Pack all the things prone to wrinkle inside out, like dresses (in plastic), and the wrinkles will be less noticeable.
8. If it's humid out, try to pack in air-conditioning, as it creates less dampness in your valise.
9. Don't bring new shoes. Walking around on a sightseeing tour and discovering that your shoes cut painfully into your foot is sheer torment.
10. Inspect every item you are packing for rips, missing buttons, or any stains.
11. Lay everything out on the bed before you put it into the suitcase; this helps you see what you have and eliminate any doubles you may have.
12. List the events you need outfits to wear to. Make sure you are covered.
13. Make sure you only travel with your style pieces! You won't feel bad wearing them more than once.

OTHER TRAVEL TIPS

1. Use a recognizable pouch for airline tickets; that way it's easy to identify in your purse or travel bag.
2. Drink one eight-ounce glass of water for every hour of flying! Plane travel dehydrates and causes headaches.
3. Save all your trial-size containers and refill them for trips.

INCIDENTALS NOT TO FORGET

• Your passport
• Calamine lotion for mosquito bites
• Avon's Skin So Soft, a great mosquito repellent

- Mini sewing kit (most hotels provide them)
- Sunscreens; buying them there is too costly
- Hairbrush, and a blow-dryer if you can't do without. Check the current in the country you're traveling to and make sure you don't need an adapter. I have a mini for travel.
- Nail polish, clear—it stops panty hose runs.
- Nail file
- A razor (it really is easier than carrying an electric)
- Tylenol (or whatever you take for a headache)
- Rolaids
- Toothpaste and toothbrush
- Perfume (save those samples of your fragrance for this)
- Moisturizer
- Deodorant or antiperspirant
- Shampoo and conditioner
- Your makeup
- A credit card (even if you insist upon paying cash, a credit card is invaluable to rent a car or a hotel room in an emergency)

Forget:

- Towels—hotels have them
- Your bulky bathrobe; carry a sleep T-shirt instead.
- One more outfit—if you really follow the above list, you'll have enough to mix for a week!

Chapter Nineteen

WHAT SIZE AM I?

INFORMATION ON SIZING

Buy the size that fits you. I don't care what size you are, and chances are no one else does either. If you gain nothing else from this section, get this: trying to squeeze yourself into a size smaller just to tell everyone that you did is uncomfortable and unflattering! Don't do it!

Don't buy for someday, buy for who you are now. Now granted, there are always exceptions to this. If you just lost sixty pounds and are in the process of taking off another twenty, that's different.

That does not include the rest of us, who are always saying, "I have to lose five pounds before I buy new clothes." If you've been at your present weight or size for more than six months, chances are you're there for a while.

And, my last word on size: I had a client once who didn't want her husband to know what size she was. He decided to buy her some clothes as a surprise. But when he went into her closet, he couldn't locate her size anywhere—because she had cut out all the size tags. It wastes energy to be ashamed of your size.

THE FOUR POPULAR SIZE CATEGORIES

There are four popular categories of sizes in America today.

Junior Sizes

Junior cuts are narrower. Yes, narrower, as in slimmer at the hips. That is why we outgrow those sizes. Very few junior vendors are expensive, because they are outgrown and out of style soon. If it's a junior, the clothes are styled and sized for a thinner and younger female.

The sizing for juniors begins in odd numbers. Sometimes they are 1/2 or 3/4 or 5/6. If they start with an odd number, they are considered junior.

Sizes for juniors:
1, 3, 5, 7, 9, 11, 13.
3–13 is the typical size range for juniors.
Also S-M-L is the size span.
S = 3–5
M = 7–9
L = 11–13

Special Sizes

It has been estimated that by the year 2000, more than 60 percent of the female population will be a special size. Presently the average American woman is 5′4″ and a size 14. Which means there are a whole lot of taller size 18s and shorter size 8s.

A special size is anyone whose body doesn't fit into the standard missy or junior size category. For years these women had to make do with styles and fabrics that were anything but fashionable.

Years ago, for the fuller-figured women, it was almost all polyester fabric in designs that were bargain-basement specials. For petites, it was a rack of clothing shoved behind missy and simply labeled petite. Often these clothes were not even fit tested by the manufacturers, with pant inseams that were anything but comfortable, and sweaters that were cut too short or too long. Special sizes have come a long way since then.

Women's sizes grew out of the budget area. Fuller-figured women demanded better clothing, and eventually, manufacturers listened. By late 1990, the women's customer no longer had to be ashamed of what she wore. Thankfully, more designers got on the bandwagon and began manufacturing clothes for the woman whose size had arrived!

Petite Sizes

The petite industry, on the other hand, grew out of better clothing. The first item to hit the floor for petites was the suit. Petites needed more casual clothes. Weekend wear was unheard of until Liz Claiborne came alone in the early 1980s. By 1985, vendors were coming out of the woodwork to manufacture petites.

Today, petites and women's departments

(in major department stores) combined take up about 13 percent of the floor space in the store, but they do almost 22 percent of the stores total volume.

Technically, petite is about proportion, while to those of us who were hemming for years it was about height (and clothes that didn't have bows and froufrou lace).

The proportion that I speak of is the distance from your bust to waist, and from waist to hip. Here's the tricky part: most manufacturers of petites will give a slightly different measurement. A petite woman is generally between ¼ and 1 inch shorter in both of these places than her missy counterpart.

> **Tip:** Petites look better if their skirt is above the knee or slightly below. Don't let your skirt cut you off in the middle of your calf. Long skirts should hit you in the bottom of the calf.
>
> **Tip:** Both petites and fuller-sizes can wear longer skirts. Above or below the calf is proper proportion.

A prime example of a petite proportion problem could be found in the anorak jacket. Petite women couldn't wear anoraks (long jackets with a drawstring at the waist) years ago, because any style that had to rest on the waist was always way too long.

Therefore, a petite woman can be up to

5′6″ if she's short enough in the middle. That is why *there is such a thing* as a taller petite. A taller petite shops the petite department when she wants a more fitted look. Although it's best for her to shop collections like Jones New York or Karen Kane, she can then find a matching piece in the missy area. Since petites are also shorter in the rise, a woman with a longer torso may find that missy pants fit her better.

Because petites are mostly the missy body type, the sizing will be even numbers. You may come across junior sizing in petites, which is why you'll see odd numbers sometimes in petites.

> **Myth:** Petites can only wear stripes that are north to south. Not true! I've seen some wonderful petite garments where the stripes traveled east to west and looked great! The key to this is proportion. If it's a petite garment, then it was meant to fit you.

> **Tip:** The proper length for a petite jacket is fingertip length. Hold your hand against your thigh. If the garment is longer than your middle finger, it's too long for you proportionally. The same is true for sweatshirts or T-shirts worn over leggings. Don't wear your tops longer than fingertip length or they will be out of proportion.

Some petite department store buyers get mad at me when they hear me tell customers that they may still have to hem their clothes. I know. It's supposed to be ready to wear. But not all of us are the perfect size, even in petites—and we may still have to alter.

Why don't they all go from 2 to 24? Too costly. In addition, a shorter size span helps keep fit problems to a minimum.

Fit is easier to control if the size run is only ten sizes. Bridge manufacturers typically begin their size runs in smaller sizes, while moderates will begin larger.

Sizes for petites:
2–12
4–14
6–16
8–18
P-S-M (sometimes L) is usually the size span.
P = 2–4
S = 6–8
M = 10–12
L = 14–16

Women's Sizing

Women's customers have their own sizing—keep in mind that it is even numbered, so for the most part it was fitted for a woman's body.

Sizes for fuller women:
14–24W (W = women's);
for petite proportions:
14–24WP (WP = women's petites)
(Some lines may begin with a 12 and go to 22)
Here are the equivalents of 1X, 2X, and 3X:
1X = 14–16
2X = 18–20
3X = 22–24
For moderate or budget, the sizing is slightly larger:
1X = 16–18
2X = 20–22
3X = 24–26

Missy Sizing

Missy sizing is everything that is not a special size or a junior. Missy can range in cost from moderate to high-priced designers. The body types for a missy are either a missy or mature. Juniors have their own sizing and category.

Missy sizing runs the same as petites; in general, the size span is from 2 to 12, or 4 to 14, or 6 to 16, or 8 to 18.

Sizes for missy:
Designers usually begin in the smaller size range:
2–12
4–14

Moderates usually begin in slightly larger sizes:

6–16
8–18

Also S-M-L is the size span.

If it's designer, the small begins in a smaller size:

S = 2–4
M = 6–8
L = 10–12

More moderate sizes begin fuller:

S = 4–6
M = 8–10
L = 12–14

Dresses sometimes will be sized in junior sizes but sold in the missy dress area. If it is a junior label, they may be appealing to the customer who has outgrown juniors. If the vendor's style is more junior, they will be sized accordingly.

The question of the hour is, how tall is a missy customer? It varies. Typically she is taller than 5'4".

In general, Italian designers tend to cut their sizes fuller, while the French tend to cut smaller. The moral of the story is that you must always try on the garment because the size on the tag may say one thing and the fit may be another.

There is a general rule that you'll be a smaller size in more expensive clothes, but don't rely upon that either, since fabrics vary.

While you may be a size 8 in cotton, you may be a 10 in linen.

THE THREE BODY TYPES USED BY MANUFACTURERS

Manufacturers fit their garments on a model who is one of three body types: junior, missy, or mature. This is unrelated to the department store categories of juniors, missy, petite, and women's.

It would be unfair of me to tell you that I created this concept myself, when in truth it was Carolyn Strauss who discovered this system along with me. We originally covered this in our book *Specialty Modeling*. I've updated it slightly.

Junior

A Junior body tends to have a more defined waist, a small bust (usually a B cup or slightly smaller), and rounded hips that are no more than two inches larger than her bust. She is the most evenly proportioned of all body types.

Many Sporty and Romantic style types tend to have a junior body as an adult. A Trendy may be a junior type too, but if she is, it's either natural or making her body "perfect" is her hobby.

Missy

A missy body will be anywhere from one to five inches thicker in the waist than her junior counterpart. Most missy types will have a B cup, while fuller figures will have a C cup. Her hips are naturally three to five inches bigger than her bust. (Aren't you relieved to see *that* on paper?) She has a full behind, thick thighs, and not much of a tummy problem.

Any style type can fall under missy.

Mature

A mature woman tends to have a fuller bust than a missy. This figure type is typically associated with an older woman, although it's not always the case. Her waist is closer in measurement to her hips. She has a flatter behind, thinner thighs, and a little bit of a tummy.

Any style type can be a mature.

(While a missy loves the fit of a trouser, a mature woman will put on a trouser and say, "Why is there so much material in here?" as she points to the seat of her pants and pulls at the excess material in the thigh area.)

WHY ARE THERE SO MANY SHOULDER PADS?

Shoulder pads are primarily used to compensate for fuller hips and make us all look proportional. Most women are fuller in the hip area, and manufacturers balance this with shoulder pads.

When a manufacturer fit tests a garment, they look to see how the outfit falls on the model. Let's say it's a sweater set—a cardigan with a matching short-sleeved sweater. They determine if the two pieces will be worn together or separately.

If the pieces are to be worn together, they may only put one set of shoulder pads in (frequently in the cardigan). If the model still looks big in the middle, they'll put in the second set. In addition, if these two pieces are designed to be worn separately, both pieces could have shoulder pads.

To experiment with this, put on an outfit with shoulder pads and remove them. Now look at your hips. If you're like most of us, your midsection will seem to get larger. That's how manufacturers determine how many sets of shoulder pads should be in an outfit.

Tip: The heavily shoulder padded look may be "out," but for a special size woman, they are very important in creating a nice proportional look.

Chapter Twenty

DECIDING WHERE TO SHOP

While style does dictate to a great degree where to shop, there are more than a few options available. Experience has taught me that we are naturally drawn to the place we feel the best shopping. Although there really is no one place that is right for each style type, because any store can appeal to all styles or just one particular style at any given time.

Let's take a look at a few options:

DEPARTMENT STORES

I love department stores. I'm a petite, and most major stores have petite departments. Since I'm also a Classic, chances are they'll have what I want. Although other style types can also find what they want easily, sometimes I have to send Trendys and Romantics to boutiques.

Department stores are set up by departments, hence the name. In general, they'll have Juniors, Clubhouse (very traditional styles), Moderate, Designers, Dresses, and Special Sizes (petites and women's sizes). There may also be several different moderate departments.

The larger the store, the more "shops" they'll have inside. Ralph Lauren is one of dozens of manufacturers with mini shops in department stores. These mini shops have proven very successful, and we're already seeing more of them.

In addition, most department stores have what's called a private label. A private label is what a store feels that they cannot get from a vendor at a reasonable price. Hence, they invent a "name" or label and fill in where they feel they need goods. A private label is exclusive to that store. The store goes to a manufacturer, sometimes a famous one, and asks them to create a line of clothes that will have the store's own label. For example, J. C. Penney's private label is called Hunt Club.

Separates are a large part of a store's inventory. Unlike designers, who put out their "collections," which are made to be worn together, separates are pieces that are sold separately to add to your wardrobe. Most department stores carry many separates.

Fashion is happening at all price points, from moderate through better, bridge, and designer. Department stores have realized that no matter what your budget, you want fashion. This is particularly true when it comes to special sizes, which were often the poor cousins to missy sizes.

Gone are the days when we went to the "designer" department to see what was "in." Today, all you need do is walk down the aisle at Dillard's or Bergner's to see the newest trends.

To see the new styles, look at what's on the mannequins. All stores have them, or at the very least displays. You can also get ideas on how to update your wardrobe this way. Sometimes something as simple as a new way to tie a scarf can update last season's outfit.

How to Shop a Department within a Department Store

Scout around for a sales associate who is your style type (or at least understands it), works in your favorite department, and then introduce yourself. Let her know you have a list and let her see it. Tell her the truth about you—your real size, your double life, how much you really want to spend. Don't be shy or reserved here. Trust me when I tell you that she's heard it all! An honest relationship with her will pay off later in phone calls that let you know that outfit you wanted just got marked down or returned in your size, or that a piece you need has just hit the floor.

Getting to know the associate in your favorite department is a wonderful way to cut down on shopping time. As she gets to know you, she'll be able to mail items directly to you.

Shopping on a Saturday is impossible. If you want to shop in a department store, stay away from weekends and lunch hours. Try taking your lunch earlier or later in the day and shop then. Also, try going evenings. Either way, go earlier in the week, since the traffic *in* the stores tends to be lighter.

We all love sales. Getting a bargain is wonderful. However, when it comes to your clothing, waiting for the sale at the end of the season may not be very cost effective. Only you can decide if having that outfit, at full price, and getting the wear out of it for the few extra months is worth it to you. Often, it is. Think about how often you'll wear it, and then think if the savings at the end of the season will be worth it.

What else does a department store offer you?

Most stores today have personal shoppers. This is a fantabulous service and one you shouldn't overlook if you get distraught over shopping.

A personal shopper knows the store better than anyone, so whatever you need, she can find it for you. It is also her job to know the latest trends, and most personal shoppers are very good at what they do. The service itself is generally free, and they will make an appointment with you to measure you and go over your needs. Most of them don't care how tight your budget is, they'll work with you to find bargains. It really is wonderful because they are in the store all the time and can find things that you might not see.

Department stores also bring in experts in their field to give seminars and host fashion shows. Designers send their representatives in to speak on their line. If you like a particular line (say, Carole Little), these representatives will tell you what's new and suggest ways to wear their newest clothes.

Return policies are great, and if you have a receipt, chances are they won't even bat an eyelash over your dissatisfaction.

Shopping department stores is fabulous because the selection is vast and you can almost always find something.

THE NATIONAL CHAIN STORES

They are inexpensive and reasonable, a great place to buy some basics. Sportbras, socks, underwear, and turtlenecks are found at considerable savings. You can often buy four turtlenecks in different colors for far less than anywhere else. Yes, you may be sacrificing quality.

However, if there's a trend that you'd like to have and you're not sure it will stay in style, by all means buy it here.

Sometimes you can find a deal on shoes, and they're quite good. If they don't feel good on your feet though, don't buy them. You can do some serious damage to your feet trying to "break them in."

J. C. Penney is an interesting alternative in this arena. They will have current fashion items that you cannot find anywhere else at prices that are reasonable. Shopping Penney's is a joy because they have such a diverse selection. And each store will vary greatly depending upon who is buying for that store. They give a great deal of leeway to their buyers, allowing them to select from a wide range of items and thus tailoring the store to the customer in that particular area. If the buyer is a Trendy, it'll be more updated; if she's a Traditional, it'll be more traditional.

Crystal Armstrong buys Women's in Torrance, California, and she is by far the best buyer I've ever come across in a Penney's store. She always manages to have an item before the trend hits, and I always find unusual items in her departments.

I would be amiss if I didn't mention the emergence of Sears as a new place to look for women's fashions. Watch Sears as an emerging new resource.

When to Shop National Chain Stores

Shop one of these stores when you need a basic, or when you want a look and aren't concerned with how long the item will last. I send clients with budget considerations to these stores.

THE SPECIAL-SIZE STORE

When Forgotten Woman hit the scene back in the 1980s, a sigh of relief came from large-size women everywhere. Soon after, it was followed by Petite Sophisticate for petites. Today there are hundreds of special-size stores nationwide.

In a special-size store, the benefit of course is that you can shop in a place where almost everything will be available in your size! You won't be tempted by what you can't have . . . and you'll get *very* personalized service.

In addition, chances are they may have a slightly different selection than the department stores at either end of the mall. Their prices are *sometimes* higher, but most often they are competitive.

However, since women's (or petites) is all they sell, they are usually quite knowledgeable about their merchandise.

THE SPECIALTY STORE

Specialty stores primarily cater to people of a particular size, style, price range, or gender, although there are unisex specialty stores, too. (The Gap and Banana Republic are two examples of unisex specialty stores.) Some stores are mini department stores. They cater to all a woman's wardrobe needs, unlike a department store, which has everything from electronics to chocolate.

The higher the price category, the more personalized the service. The idea behind a specialty store is that you will find things that are unique. While they are not meant to be discounters, hopefully, it'll be affordable too.

The Gap enjoyed some renewed success in the early 1990s when Gap style became mainstream. That's easy to understand. Any style type could wear their clothes, and they were very easy to put together and looked good.

As soon as Gap hit its peak, The Limited came on strong. (Lane Bryant, L'Express, Victoria's Secret, and The Limited are all owned by one company.) Both The Limited and L'Express are very popular. Why? Think about how many style types can wear what is hanging in their windows.

Don't miss the opportunity to walk a mall near you and make mental notes as to what style types are featured in the store windows. This may tell you why you haven't shopped in a particular store before—the style they are appealing to isn't yours!

Stores like Marshall's, Loehman's, and Ross are discounters. Shopping in any of these stores takes patience. You have to be willing to leave without a purchase if need be. They're hard to shop, but you can find some wonderful things, *if* you're willing to be flexible but not gullible. Remember that a bargain is no bargain if you don't wear it.

If you don't like something, return it. But keep your receipts! Without a receipt most stores won't give a cash refund. There are too many people today who shoplift and then try and return the goods.

> **Tip:** Ask what day new merchandise is put on the floor. Shopping the day of a new shipment is ideal for a wider selection.

THE BOUTIQUE

Although boutiques fall into the category of specialty stores, I want to mention them separately. Boutiques are popular haunts for many a Trendy, Dramatic, and Romantic. Other style types may shop them too, but you can find many one-of-a-kind items at a good boutique, which is not as big a consideration for a Traditional, Classic, or Sporty.

Price is not a consideration at a boutique, as many of them are pricey. But the one-of-a-kind items you can find, make it worth it.

THE CATALOG

I love catalog shopping. Bargains or Convenience? Sometimes both, but not always. Bargains are not what catalogs are about; there are some that are discounters, though. Catalogs are primarily for convenience.

Catalogs are usually great places for basics and weekend wear. Here is mini list of a few catalogs and style types they cater to:

Traditional:
Talbots   (800) 888-5268
Carroll Reed   (800) 343-5770
Newport News   (800) 688-2830
Lord & Taylor   (800) 223-7440

Sporty
Eddie Bauer   (800) 645-7467 (Traditional and Trendy too)
J Crew   (800) 562-0258 (Traditional, Classic, and Trendy too)
Allen, Allen USA   (800) 422-0466 (Classic and Trendy too)

Classic
Clifford & Wills   (800) 922-0114
Neiman Marcus by mail   (800) 634-6267

All Types
Victoria's Secret   (800) 888-8200
One 212   (800) 216-2221

WHAT TO WEAR TO SHOP IN

Comfort is very important! Wear comfortable shoes. However, I suggest that if you are shopping for a specific suit or dress, bring the shoes you plan to wear with the outfit. This way, if you find the pant or skirt you're looking for and it needs an alteration, you can alter it to work with the shoes it'll be worn with.

WHOM SHOULD YOU SHOP WITH?

Ideally, your own style type is best to shop with. If that's not possible, then the type opposite you is a wonderful choice. Your opposite and you know instantly when something isn't right for the other and can easily spot the other choices.

I do suggest not shopping with the style type after you if they intimidate you; if not, then just make sure that you're not buying what they like for you instead of what's right for you.

MAKE THAT LIST AND BUY IT!

Don't be afraid to buy what you need. You've made your list. You know what you need. Now go get it!

Chapter Twenty-One

YOU ARE READY!

I've always felt that in fashion, if real folks don't understand something then it's not worth doing. I searched for myself for a long time, and it was in finding and wearing my proper style that I have felt most at home. It is my sincere wish that you too have found this to be simple and fun.

What did your "style" reveal to you? Is there an accent that you liked and would like to try out? Perhaps you want to play with a new color on your wheel; choose one that reflects best what you want to say and watch how others respond to you.

I've enjoyed working with you. Perhaps I'll be blessed with meeting you someday at one of my seminars. Until then, I'll leave you with . . .

My best wishes,
Tori